15-MINUTE REIKI

This excellent book is holistic in the very truest sense. Not only dealing in the most informative way with the fascinating subject of Reiki, it also acts as an indispensable workbook to aid self-development. It is suited to practitioners of every level of Reiki as well as complete beginners and it is a book I shall turn to time and again.
Professor Jayne Goddard, President, Complementary Medical Association

Everyone has the ability to become a healer, of both themselves and others. The practice of Reiki has dramatically changed my life, and the lives of all who have practised or received this lovely, healing energy. In *15-Minute Reiki*, Chris and Penny Parkes easily show the advantages of practising Reiki for as little as 15 minutes a day. I would highly endorse it!
Dawna Walter, Reiki Master and presenter of The Life Laundry

What a great book! When the clock is ticking, this book actually teaches you how to find the time for Reiki. *15-Minute Reiki* is an important book for anyone already interested in Reiki and a must for anyone considering training.
Lawrence Ellyard, author of Reiki Healer

This book shows you how Reiki can enhance your life. It contains many self-empowerment tools for happy, healthy, harmonious living. Chris and Penny Parkes are Reiki Masters/teachers and life coaches as well.
Tanmaya Honervogt, International Reiki Master-Teacher

Parallel with conventional medicine, Reiki is a wonderful tool for healing yourself and others. Chris and Penny Parkes show you how you can use it to transform your life. As well as treating all kinds of physical conditions, you learn how to eliminate energy drains, harness your inner power, nurture your spiritual well-being and live the life of your dreams. Read it and be inspired.
Uri Geller

15-Minute Reiki is a necessary reminder of how to integrate Reiki into our busy lives. Chris and Penny show how easy, simple, and helpful it is to use Reiki's very profound gift.
Kimberly Fleisher, Founder, The Reiki School and Clinic of Philadelphia

15-Minute Reiki is highly recommended to anyone considering Reiki training and to practitioners at all levels. Although Reiki must be experienced to be fully understood, this book deals effectively with a variety of questions that can arise. The written exercises can be used by anyone to improve their life.
Kathryn Mannyng, Certified Reiki Practitioner and Musician of Minnesota

15-MINUTE
REIKI

HEALTH AND HEALING AT YOUR FINGERTIPS

Chris and Penny Parkes

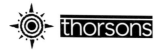

Thorsons
An Imprint of HarperCollins *Publishers*
77–85 Fulham Palace Road
Hammersmith, London W6 8JB

The website address is: www.thorsonselement.com

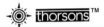

and *Thorsons*
are trademarks of HarperCollins *Publishers* Limited

First published 2004

10 9 8 7 6 5 4 3 2 1

A percentage of the royalties from this book
are donated to the charity Children with Aids.

Photography by Guy Hearn
Illustrations © PCA Creative Design

A catalogue record of this book is
available from the British Library

ISBN 0 00 715891 2

Printed and bound in Great Britain by
Martins the Printers Ltd, Berwick upon Tweed

For Yvette
whose courage and positive outlook are
an inspiration to all who know her

Contents

PART IV: REIKI TRAINING COURSES

PART V: RESOURCES

Introduction

A day is a miniature eternity.
RALPH WALDO EMERSON

Many people have told us they would love to include Reiki in their lives, but there simply wasn't the time. If there were, there wasn't the energy, the space, the motivation or the know-how to make Reiki a meaningful and inspiring part of everyday living. If this sounds familiar, then this book is written for you.

Would you like more harmony, less stress and more balance in your life? Well, you're not alone. Many people are tired of fast-paced, fragmented lifestyles and are interested in a more meaningful life with time for reflection and energy to invest in physical, emotional and spiritual well-being.

Whether you are a stressed-out executive, a student, a home-worker, someone juggling a busy home life with a career, or someone who is continually tired – with the help of Reiki you can make positive changes. We will share with you many ways to overcome the obstacles that prevent you living a fulfilling life.

Reiki is a wonderfully simple, hands-on healing art. It is an effective method of relaxation and stress-relief. It restores harmony, increases vitality and can treat almost any ailment.

It is our intention to pass on some tools to heal yourself and become the perfect healer that you intrinsically are. Reiki can enable you to take charge of your own health and well-being. Using the various techniques, you will discover the many benefits of this extraordinary and fascinating energy medicine.

Wishing you well in your quest to understand the mystery and beauty of life through the use of Reiki.

IN LOVE AND LIGHT

CHRIS AND PENNY PARKES

How to Use this Book

15-Minute Reiki is divided into four sections to make it practical, easy to use and straightforward to read.

Part One helps you get a feel for Reiki by explaining what it is and how you can use it. Even if you are already an experienced practitioner or a teacher of Reiki, it also includes new information and an updated history of its origins.

Part Two illustrates how Reiki can be used to treat specific illnesses or injuries, even when time is limited. It contains useful information on a range of ailments, from everyday complaints to chronic conditions and first aid. For the Reiki practitioner it contains special ways to treat specific imbalances. This part can be read a little at a time or used for reference when required. In addition, there are tips to keep you healthy, strong and less susceptible to illness.

Part Three puts the theory into action, with exercises for self-healing and transformation. It includes strategies that will enable you to bring more energy, balance and harmony into your life, so you can harness your inner power and live your dreams.

Part Four describes the different levels of Reiki training, and includes lots of practical guidance. It includes answers to frequently asked questions such as how to find the right teacher and how to become a practitioner. For those who have taken Reiki training, it covers new ground and suggests creative ways of using it.

While Reiki is in essence a straightforward healing art, each person will develop his or her own way of relating to it. This book is designed to be an accessible guide to enable Reiki to fit in with your life, rather than the other way around.

PART ONE

1 Origins of Reiki Healing

Guard well your spare moments. They are like uncut diamonds.
Discard them and their value will never be known. Improve
them and they will become the brightest gems in a useful life.
RALPH WALDO EMERSON

The word 'Reiki' refers to a simple, hands-on healing technique discovered by Dr Mikao Usui in Japan in the early 1900s. Its popularity has spread all over the world, particularly throughout America and Western Europe.

Dr Usui called this energy medicine Reiki, meaning 'life-force energy'. It describes a process of healing that is brought about through the use of hands laid on the body in certain positions. This healing art is passed from teacher to student by a series of mystic attunements that are carried out during a Reiki training course.

The empowerments help each person to open up to and receive an increased amount of life-force energy. As the energetic amplification varies at each stage, the study of Reiki is divided up into three levels or degrees.

In quantum physics, energy is recognized as the fundamental substance of which the universe is composed. Our physical universe, while seeming solid, is actually composed of densely vibrating energy particles. All these particles vibrate at different speeds, and their speed holds the pattern of their physical form. Physicists describe particles not as isolated grains of matter, but as interconnections in an inseparable cosmic web.

Our own physical bodies are composed of energy. Everything within and around us is, too. The various parts of the body are made up of energy patterns. These patterns have many different forms and densities. These forms can remain constant or be subject to change. Some alter quickly and easily. An example of this is human thought. Other forms of energy take more time to change, such as human tissue. Denser energy forms, such as rocks, take much longer to change, yet even these can be altered by a lighter, finer energy, such as water, though this occurs over a very long period.

As well as being composed of energy, we also have energy running through us. Many Eastern forms of medicine believe this flow of energy sustains life itself. Universal life force energy is said to pass through the body via channels or an energetic grid, known as 'meridians'. In Chinese medicine, the aim of acupuncture is to stimulate the flow of energy through these pathways.

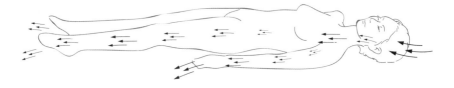

While we are healthy and strong, there is a powerful flow of energy running through the body. When we are feeling stressed or unwell, this flow of energy is reduced. Reiki is a simple and effective way of restoring the flow. In time and with practice, it is possible to achieve vibrant health, inner calm, balance and harmony.

It is now known that Reiki is the secularized form of a much more complex system of spiritual healing techniques developed by Dr Usui. He designed the system to be accessible to people of all backgrounds. While it is not necessary for a practitioner to believe in Reiki's more mystical element, it does require regular practice to reap the maximum benefit.

While spontaneous cures have been known and chronic conditions eased, Reiki is at its most effective when used frequently as a preventative measure and to speed up post-operative healing. Regular use calms the mind, relaxes the body and soothes the soul.

Overall, it is a gentle, non-invasive way of keeping healthy and staying relaxed. Its regular use can enable you to bring joy, peace and vitality into your life.

WHY LEARN REIKI?

Having taught Reiki for many years, it was apparent to us that it is one of the simplest yet most profound healing systems. We have had the honour of witnessing many individual transformations that have occurred through its use.

At the beginning of each course, we ask participants why they have decided to study Reiki. The answers vary. Many tell us their decision followed a spontaneous healing or a particular state of consciousness experienced during a treatment. Others noticed positive changes in their friends or partners following a course. There are many personal reasons, but mostly it is because they want to make a difference both to their own lives and to others'.

The following are some of the reasons why people have chosen to take Reiki training:

- It is easy to learn by anyone, regardless of background, age or experience.
- Reiki enhances physical, mental, emotional and spiritual well-being.
- Reiki is a natural, drug free healing remedy.
- Reiki calms the nervous system and is a natural antidote to stress.
- Reiki can be used anywhere, at any time.
- Reiki promotes self-reliance and can be used effectively as a self-treatment.
- Reiki relieves physical symptoms and works towards alleviating their underlying cause.
- Reiki raises self-awareness.
- Reiki combines well with other healing modalities.

- Reiki can be used effectively with children, animals and plants.
- Reiki promotes inner peace and calm by dissolving the barriers to harmony.
- Reiki can be used alongside allopathic (orthodox) medicine and medical treatments.
- Reiki can be used to solve problems and achieve goals.
- You don't have to believe in Reiki for it to work.
- The benefits last a lifetime.

2 The History of Reiki

Reiki is new to the West although its origins stretch back to the latter part of nineteenth-century Japan, when its founder, Mikao Usui, was born on 15 August 1865.

Usui was born into a privileged class. He was highly educated, graduating with a doctorate in literature. He also spoke several languages and was knowledgeable on subjects such as medicine, philosophy and theology. Although he was a practising Buddhist, his memorial stone says that he was also well versed in Taoism and Christian scriptures. He read widely and travelled extensively overseas. Usui is believed to have studied both Japanese and Chinese healing techniques.

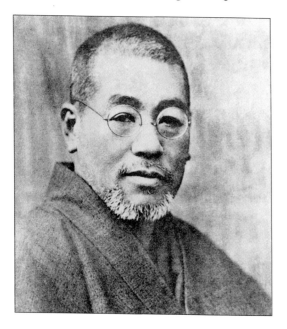

Usui married and had two children. He went into business whilst continuing to study medicine and spirituality in his spare time. This led him to become involved with a Buddhist group who had a centre located at the foot of Mount Kurama Yama. He began to conduct his own extensive research, much of which was undertaken in the libraries and monasteries of Kyoto. He learned many healing arts and in time became a knowledgeable and respected teacher. He taught many ways to treat the illnesses that were sweeping through Japan at that time. He also practised meditation and would regularly go on intense retreats for both solitude and spiritual development. Whilst on one particular retreat on Mount Kurama, he had an unusual experience which changed the course of his life.

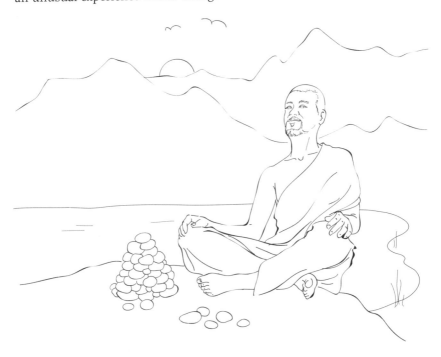

It was during the early hours of his last morning on the mountain that he noticed a light in the dark sky. It seemed to be moving rapidly towards him. He was unsure whether to move out of the way. He decided to remain, even though he knew this was risky. The light came closer and seemed to hit his forehead. He began to see strange symbols appearing before his eyes. He became aware of information being imparted to him, as each symbol came into view. By the time the revelation ended, daylight was breaking and Usui found himself once again alone on the mountain.

He knew he had received insight into a powerful healing method. This was an exciting moment for him. Feeling energized and elated, he made his way down the mountain and returned to Kyoto. After assimilating the knowledge, Usui went on to develop it into a practical and accessible healing art. He first started practising on those closest to him, then began to offer treatments to those in need and to teach his new healing method to his students. In 1921, Usui opened a clinic in Tokyo and began to teach Reiki for the first time.

On 1 September 1923, a devastating earthquake ripped through Tokyo. Over 140,000 people died. Another 40,000 were killed when a fire tornado swept in from across the sea. Three million homes were destroyed. The city was in shock, with the collapse of public amenities such as water and sewers. Countless people were injured or homeless. Over 50,000 people suffered serious injuries.

Usui and his students offered Reiki to many people. In February 1924, he built a new larger clinic outside Tokyo to handle the throng of patients. Usui's fame spread all over Japan. The Emperor honoured him for the way in which he and his students helped the victims of the earthquake. Many people wanted to learn Usui's healing method, and to meet demand he began teaching a more simplified form.

In May 1925, a retired naval officer, Chirjiro Hayashi, became a student of Usui. He had studied with him for only nine months when Usui unexpectedly suffered a stroke and died. Hayashi remained with Usui's school until 1931, when he left to set up his own clinic in Tokyo. Hayashi modified the system, creating a number of degrees to represent the different levels of learning, and also developed a more complex set of hand positions suitable for clinical use.

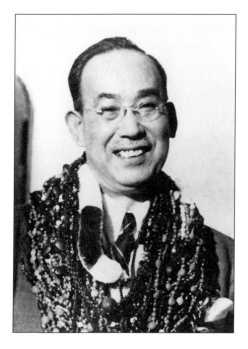

Although Reiki is still taught and practised in Japan today, it was through Dr Hayashi that the knowledge of Reiki came to the West. The transition occurred after Hayashi treated a Japanese-American, Mrs Hawayo Takata.

Mrs Takata lived in Hawaii with her husband and two young daughters. When her husband died at only 34 years old, her health began to suffer. It continued to deteriorate and some five years later, she decided to return to Japan for a series of operations. Before the first one took place, she heard a voice telling her the operation was unnecessary. After making further enquiries about alternatives to surgery, Mrs Takata was directed to attend Dr Hayashi's clinic.

Mrs Takata was initially sceptical, having no prior knowledge or experience of Reiki. She was curious to know why such heat was being generated by the practitioner's hands and demanded to know where electrical machinery was being hidden. Dr Hayashi explained the basic concepts of

Reiki to satisfy her curiosity. She returned daily to the clinic and after several weeks, began to feel much better. In time, Mrs Takata successfully regained her health.

Following her treatment, Mrs Takata enthusiastically applied to become a student of Dr Hayashi. She was told that the technique was not taught to foreigners. After convincing him of her commitment, Dr Hawashi eventually relented.

Whilst living at his home, studying and practising at his clinic, Mrs Takata trained to be a practitioner. She returned to Hawaii in 1937. Dr. Hayashi followed her several weeks later with his daughter. He is believed to have stayed for several months to help build her practice. Before returning to Japan, he initiated her as a teacher or Master. Two years later, on 10 May 1940, Dr Hayashi died, having passed his knowledge on to a number of his Japanese students in addition to Mrs Takata, who is believed to have been the last Master he taught.

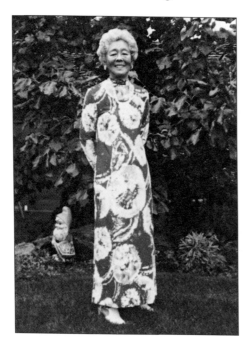

It wasn't until the early 1970s that Reiki found its way to the West, when Mrs Takata left her home in Hawaii for mainland America. Before her death in December 1979, she had initiated 22 teachers. Each was taught on a one-to-one basis.

Following her death, it was not clear who should succeed her. Two of Mrs Takata's 22 students claimed to be her sole successor. Barbara Weber Ray declared that Mrs Takata, who had passed on all seven degrees exclusively to her, had appointed her. Meanwhile Mrs Takata's granddaughter, Phyllis Furomoto, stated that she alone was the true successor and the knowledge was contained within the three levels she taught.

The Reiki Masters who supported Phyllis Furomoto arranged a second meeting. They agreed to standardize the teaching and subsequently the Reiki Alliance was formed. Since that time, the Alliance has worked hard to encourage the international Reiki community to come into alignment with their understanding and views of the Usui System of Natural Healing.

Barbara Weber Ray believes her system to be more authentic as it contained extra knowledge given to her by Mrs Takata. She went on to write the first book on Reiki, *The Reiki Factor*. Her system became known as the Radiance Technique. Mrs Takata's system is the best known today with millions of Practitioners worldwide.

REIKI TODAY

Since Mrs Takata's death, these two systems have been taught in a consistent way. More recently, numerous variations have been created. Differing from the traditional methods, these techniques have their own approach. Whether they have a legitimate lineage, a sound methodology or are a marketing ploy is a matter for the discerning. There are far too many in number to comment on here.

Both Dr Usui and Dr Hayashi trained a number of their students to teach Reiki. It has evolved quite differently in Japan, where it continues to be taught today.

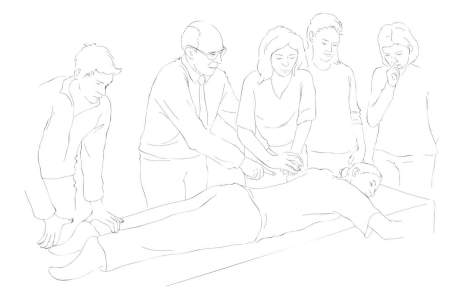

A number of people have attempted to research and compile a detailed history of the life and teachings of Dr Usui, from mainly Japanese sources. The history is difficult to research as material considered sacred in Japan is protected from those not entitled to access it. Attempts have met with only partial success, resulting in new revelations emerging on a regular basis. Furthermore, a number of key sources are no longer living, making it very difficult to distinguish between legend and fact.

The discovery of Dr Usui's memorial and the establishment of links to Japanese Reiki Schools in the early 1990s have revealed some differences in the way that Reiki has evolved in Japan. Since stories about Dr Usui's healing quest were handed down orally, it was inevitable that the contents would change over time. As far as individual techniques are concerned, the Japanese and Western method of teaching Reiki are broadly similar, but have a different emphasis. As a result, different exercises are taught, none better or worse than each other. Further details on Japanese Reiki techniques can be found on the website of The International House of Reiki at www.reiki.net.au.

There are now many offshoots of Dr Usui's teachings both in Japan and in the West. The essence of Dr Usui's healing art is present in all its variations. He envisaged Reiki as easy to learn, straightforward to use and effective. Having no barriers, it can reach all religions, races and cultures regardless of whether people are rich, poor, strong, weak, young or old. After a turbulent adolescence, it is evident that as it matures, Reiki is becoming a great leveller, bringing back simplicity and unity to people everywhere.

Those wishing to read more about the history of Reiki can find more detailed information in *The Reiki Sourcebook* by Bronwen and Frans Stiene or in the history section on Lawrence Ellyard's website www.taoofreiki.com.

If you have never experienced Reiki, then we hope you will be inspired to find out for yourself what it feels like, as even the best description and most illuminating historical perspective cannot compare with your own experience.

3 The Five Principles of Reiki

In order to change a person's situation in life, there has to be a change in attitude. Knowing this, Dr Usui developed five principles to help improve the quality of a person's life. These principles form an important part of the healing process at the heart of Reiki. Dr Usui had come to realize how much more powerful and effective treatment was – for the practitioner and the recipient – if these principles were adhered to. Dr Usui knew how vital it was for a person to be involved in his or her own healing process and, through these principles, he was able to inspire meaningful change.

These principles are just as relevant today as when Dr Usui developed them:

1. JUST FOR TODAY, DO NOT WORRY

Being unconcerned with the future, accepting of the past, and
content in the right now, is true happiness ...
HARUSAMI

Dr Usui knew that a great deal of energy can be wasted on negative trains of thought. He also knew that negative thoughts are unhelpful and likely to affect the outcome of any treatment. He reminded people that there is a divine purpose to everything, and that energy used for worrying can be more usefully employed elsewhere.

We live in a responsive universe. As long as we are able to clarify our heart's desires, our needs will be met. By trusting in the outcome we are allowing the universe to make it all possible. Our freed-up minds can then open to intuitive messages and guidance. This can take us closer to our goals or, conversely, can point to new directions offering interesting alternatives.

Sometimes, when a situation is beyond our control, a detached perspective can be invaluable and can render a desperate situation into an unexpected opportunity. One of our students, Cathy, had set her intent on finding an exciting job. She was overjoyed when an opportunity came up and she was invited for interview. On the way there, Cathy missed the train and knew the delay would mean she was unlikely to be considered. On the journey home, she had the good fortune to be sitting next to a Chief Executive in the same industry. She enjoyed talking to him, and the conversation led to her being offered a position with his company at nearly twice the salary. In addition ... she later became his wife!

A wise sage once remarked that if you are given lemons .... make lemonade. Dr Usui would undoubtedly agree.

Releasing Worry

Complete the following exercise.

1. Make a list of all the things that concern you, both personally and globally.
2. On another sheet of paper, draw 2 circles, one inside the other.
3. Inside the inner circle, list all worries or concerns that directly affect you. Include ones you can do something about. For example, 'I worry about the faulty light switch outside the bathroom.'
4. In the outer circle, write all the concerns that you cannot change. For example, whether your teenage daughter may or may not injure herself on a skiing holiday.
5. Immediately release from your thoughts everything from the outer circle. They are beyond your control, and no amount of worrying will bring any change to those situations.
6. Look at the inner circle. Can you take appropriate action so these concerns are released from your thoughts? Can an electrician be called in to mend that faulty switch?

7. Relax, knowing you have taken the necessary action, and trust that everything will work out the way you want it to.

2. JUST FOR TODAY, DO NOT BE ANGRY

When we do something out of great love rather than great expectation, more comes back to us than we could have ever imagined.
ANONYMOUS

Anger creates disharmony within the body. By asking us not to become angry, Dr Usui was not suggesting people deny their feelings. Instead, he was inviting them to respond with love.

When a situation does not live up to our expectations, we become angry. The ego doesn't like it if things don't work out as we anticipate. When inappropriately expressed, however, anger can be a very destructive emotion.

When we are aware of our reactions and are in control, this can be a learning experience and a powerful motivator for change. Instead of stopping anger, observe it. Be aware and focus on it in a detached way, without judgement. Eventually, its energy field will dissipate.

Anger with awareness can powerfully affect outcomes. A loving response without anger can transform a situation.

RELEASING ANGER

- Next time you are angry, observe it and notice the underlying fear that has caused it to surface.
- Allow yourself to feel the anger. Don't repress it. By focusing on it with awareness, the sting is taken out of it.
- If you feel yourself exploding with anger, take a brisk walk or lock yourself away and beat a pillow to release the tension. You'll be amazed how much better you feel.

3. EARN YOUR LIVING HONESTLY

The best measure of a man's honesty isn't his income tax
return. It's the zero adjust on his bathroom scale.
ARTHUR C. CLARKE

This principle is about being true to yourself and honest in your dealings with others. It is about choosing a vocation that helps you to grow and provides you with a sense of fulfilment.

When you are aligned fully to your life's purpose, you are earning your living honestly, utilizing your creativity in a way that honours who you are and enriches those around you. It allows you to meet your needs and speak your truth.

As only your heart can tell you what is most appropriate, you must listen carefully when it whispers. Everything is far less complicated when we are true to ourselves.

Being Honest With Yourself

Take a few moments to answer the following questions:

- What are you putting up with at the moment?
- What things are frustrating you about your work?
- If this week were your last week on earth, would you be happy with how you are spending your time?
- If you were being true to yourself, what would you be doing right now, personally and professionally?

4. JUST FOR TODAY, SHOW GRATITUDE TO EVERY LIVING THING

The difference between living a life of passion and adventure or living a life of pain and chaos ... is in your perception.
HARUSAMI

By reflecting on what makes our lives special, we can begin to appreciate just what brings us joy. By expressing gratitude, we can begin to understand how incredible life is, in all its diversity.

If you took a moment each day to encourage the feeling of gratitude to expand within you, a powerful inner shift would occur and bring wonderment into your life. An attitude of gratitude takes you from victim to victorious. It frees you up from the past and turns all your negatives into positives.

Gratitude seems magnetically to attract abundance, and brings more good things your way. Whenever you feel overwhelmed, allow yourself to remember the aspects of your life you have gratitude for. Don't be afraid to show it, either. When you feel and express gratitude, success, happiness and prosperity will flow into your life.

The Attitude of Gratitude

Every day, write down five things you are grateful for. It can be gratitude for your education or family. It can be anything from the beauty of a sunset to the precious moments spent with loved ones.

1. I have gratitude for:

....

....

....

....

2. Express gratitude when things go well – and maintain it even when they do not.

3. Enjoy the miracle of life and the miracle that uniquely is you.

5. JUST FOR TODAY, I WILL BE KIND AND RESPECTFUL TO ALL OF CREATION

Kindness is more important than wisdom,
and the recognition of this is the beginning of wisdom.
THEODORE ISAAC RUBIN

Man's inhumanity to his fellow man and to the environment has caused many humanitarian and ecological problems. Dr Usui appreciated that our growth and survival depends on loving actions and respect for one another and all living things.

A starting point would be to begin to view everything and everyone around you in a non-judgemental way. More importantly, the most caring action you can take is to put yourself first, because so often we don't.

By choosing to put yourself first, you begin to make decisions from a perspective of self-love. It can involve and choosing new ways to live, so you can achieve a better balance between work and family life.

Making self-love your priority allows you to observe those around you in a different way, too. It involves taking positive action and responding with warmth and compassion. By being kind and respectful to yourself, it is easier to view the world with a loving heart. When you do, the world responds. It becomes a truly wonderful place to be.

Practise Self-Love

1. *Make a list of all the things you have done that you are proud of.*
2. *Ask yourself what your life would be like if you respected or liked yourself more.*
3. *Know that you are an incredible human being. Make a list of all the things that make you special. Keep the list in a safe place, and add to it later on.*
4. *Right here, right now, make the decision to start loving yourself. There's no time to lose.*
5. *Imagine your heart filled to the brim with kindness and love. Radiate this out to those around you.*

We found that focusing on these principles was a powerful step on our own journey. They lead to a more positive outlook. Integrating them into your life is not only helpful for your Reiki practice but also develops you as a person.

Be creative. Find ways to focus on one principle at a time. In addition to the above exercises, write the principles out and place one in a prominent position each week to keep it at the forefront of your mind. Bringing the principles into your life allows gradual shifts to occur and paves the way for meaningful change.

4 How We First Came Across Reiki – by Penny Parkes

Everyone should carefully observe which way his heart draws him, and then choose that way with all his strength.
HASIDIC SAYING

There are moments in everyone's life when the world is viewed different-ly, as if for the first time. Sometimes it is because you reach a crossroads and are forced to make a radically different choice. It can happen because of choices others have made. Other times, an unexpected occurrence affects you so profoundly you know that, right up until that moment, you looked at yourself and never knew who you were or what mattered. At times like this, you feel as if you have awoken. Everything becomes clear.

My earliest and first memory of a life-changing realization came when I was about 17. I have long forgotten the circumstances that surrounded it, but the awareness has always stayed with me. I realized that the greatest tragedy of a lifetime was not to follow your heart and to live forever with regret.

The credit for this realization belongs to my mother, whose positive thinking was inspirational. I can still hear her saying 'It's always the things you don't do, that you regret.' Despite the fact that her life had more chal-lenges than most, she spent more time helping others than being saved. She practised positive thinking long before the phrase was coined. No mat-ter how challenging her days became, she continued to make the most of her life and encouraged her family, friends and colleagues to do the same. Even when faced with the prospect of her own death, she merely paused, took a deep breath and considered how many people she loved. My moth-er reflected on how lucky her life had been. She then went on to make the best use of the time she had left.

I was fortunate to grow up believing anything was possible, and later on began to read widely on the subject of self-development. When Chris and I met, we both quickly realized that while our backgrounds were different, we had much in common. Human potential fascinated us both. We attended philosophy lectures drawn from both Eastern and Western teachings. We read books on subjects such as psychology, spirituality and Eastern mysticism. We took part in a number of courses and joined various groups. We were fortunate in finding excellent teachers who provided us with encouragement and inspiration.

Being keen advocates of a holistic lifestyle, we enjoyed a nutritious diet, supplemented by vitamins and minerals. We used complementary therapies wherever possible and, additionally, Chris believed that good health depended on regular exercise. All our cupboards were filled with eco-friendly products. We ran a business that had been family owned for several generations, had three well-balanced children, supportive parents plus brothers and sisters all living nearby with their families. We were happy, healthy and blissfully unaware of what was to come.

For the two of us as a couple, the year 1991 was the catalyst for fundamental change. We were presented with a number of challenges, both personally and professionally, that led us to review our priorities and values. Our family business failed. Chris' parents became terminally ill. We were the subjects of legal action. Our health deteriorated, and each day seemed to be a feat of survival. The relationship with everyone and everything in our lives changed. We no longer knew whom we could depend upon or trust, and felt as if we had been catapulted head-first into a life to which we didn't belong. For a time, everything we had learned seemed distant and out of focus.

In the space of 12 months, our lives changed completely. Chris remembers feeling as if he had been crushed and broken into little pieces that were scattered all over the floor. He blamed himself for the loss of several hundred jobs, as well as our own livelihood. Despite all we had learned and our positive 'no pain, no gain' attitude and 'can do' perspective, it was as if we were looking at ourselves, who we were and where we were going, for the first time ever.

It was in Chris' darkest hour that I knew without any shadow of doubt that none of this mattered at all. We both knew. It just marked the end of an era, and a new beginning was just a step away. I remembered the words of Helen Keller, who said that sometimes when you are looking so hard at the door that had closed, you don't even notice that another one has opened. We began to climb out of the abyss.

One of the year's saddest events was losing both of Chris' parents within a short period. We witnessed their struggle against cancer without really being able to help, at least not in any meaningful way. Even if their deaths were inevitable, we had longed to find a way of helping them. We wondered how to ease their inner anguish other than attending to their physical needs and pain-management.

Not long after Chris' parents had passed away, my mother was diagnosed with lymphoma. While she was positive and even philosophical about the illness, we knew there must be some way in which she could be helped. It was at this point we realized how much we needed to address our own self-healing.

We read about Reiki in a magazine from the local health food shop. An American called Carrlyn Clay was visiting from Arizona and she was giving a talk on a healing art that anyone could learn. It was called Reiki. We attended out of curiosity.

The talk was fascinating. During the evening we were invited to experience a demonstration of Reiki. This turned out to be particularly interesting, as both of us had an unusual experience. A powerful feeling of love and connection to all living things overwhelmed Chris. I experienced an extraordinary feeling of peace, as if all was just as it should be.

We met Carrlyn after the talk. She was a warm, caring person whom we both immediately liked. Things happened quickly after this. We cancelled our weekend arrangements and took First-degree Reiki training instead.

Carrlyn was an excellent teacher and the course was fascinating. We had some interesting experiences while training, but no confirmation of just how effective Reiki was. Would it work for us? Would it work for others? We were shortly to find out.

We often spend time in a delightful, unspoilt seaside village called Aberdaron, in the heart of North Wales. It is a special place, serenely located in a beautiful Welsh valley, by the sea. While returning from one particular visit, we stopped briefly at a motorway service station. While there, I twisted my ankle. It swelled up and became painful. Hobbling back to the car, I sat down and steeled myself for what I anticipated would be an uncomfortable journey.

Suddenly we looked at each other. Could Reiki help? Chris put his hands gently over the area and allowed the energy to flow. To my astonishment, the pain eased after just a few minutes. Then the swelling began to subside and mobility returned. Within 20 minutes I was not only feeling fine, but I was driving again! It felt marvellous.

As soon as we got home we wanted everyone to experience this wonderful energy! Anyone who happened to have an ache or pain was offered a demonstration. We took every opportunity to try out our newly discovered healing technique.

One of the first people to receive a longer treatment was my mother. The cancer had advanced quite rapidly by this time, but she was keen to try this unusual and mysterious healing art.

While she was a positive person, she was also pragmatic and not particularly drawn to the ethereal. We knew that, whatever her experience, she could be relied upon for honest feedback. She slept deeply during the treatment and we wondered if she would remember anything at all.

When she awoke, she told us that she had experienced vivid, colourful dreams that made her feel peaceful and calm. We noticed how relaxed she looked and how her eyes seemed to sparkle again. She told us that the pain and fear had gone. She felt energized and relaxed. The strain was gone from her face.

We went on to give her regular treatments. Although she sadly died several months later, she told us how much she had benefited from the sessions. She had found the inner peace that had so eluded Chris' parents.

We went on to practise on others, and found Reiki to be effective. As soon as we were able, we took the next level, Second Degree. This was even more powerful.

It was not long afterwards that we decided to train as Reiki teachers or Masters. The apprentice-style training was intense and we came to realize the true vastness of Reiki. Everything we had ever learned and experienced came together in a way we had never dreamed of. A whole new world opened. We learned many fascinating processes which changed our lives for the better. Over time, the true secrets of Reiki were gradually revealed.

We would like to share these with you so that you can take charge of your own well-being and transform your life.

WHY WE FORMED THE REIKI SCHOOL

We are passionate about Reiki and believe that it can bring positive change. At the time we learned, classes were taught in the traditional manner, with adequate time in between each level to give students time to integrate what they had been taught. We find this is the best way of learning Reiki.

In recent years many different styles have emerged, with teachers creating their own attunements and symbols. Courses have become shorter, with two or more levels condensed and taught in a single weekend. We both came to feel that it was time to form a school where the standards were consistently high and in keeping with Dr Usui's original form.

It was important to honour the historic system of Reiki while adapting its practice to suit the needs of a modern lifestyle. Our aim is to teach creative, informative courses that hold true to Dr Usui's original vision.

We set up the Reiki School to provide the opportunity for students to receive a high standard of training so that Reiki can be used effectively for self-healing and healing others. Our classes are traditional and up to date. Those seeking a treatment can expect a proficient service from an experienced practitioner. We constantly strive to improve our courses and provide tuition dedicated to the pursuit of healing and self-improvement.

5 Time for Reiki, Time for You

Reiki can be effective, even when time is limited. While a full treatment is ideal, even just 15 minutes can make a significant difference. One of our practitioners gives Reiki to office personnel on a regular basis. They only have a short period of time and are invariably stressed. Most of them receive Reiki for about 10 to 15 minutes, usually during a lunch break. They frequently report feeling calm, alert and energized for the rest of the day.

We would like to share with you some special moments when our hearts have been touched by the healing of others.

GARY'S STORY

Each year we exhibit at our local Mind, Body & Spirit Exhibition. People are able to experience Reiki first hand. The conditions are far from ideal. Despite being noisy and crowded, however, it is possible to enjoy a blissful experience in just a few minutes.

On one busy afternoon, Gary came up to the stand. He had returned several times during the day, awaiting an opportunity to experience a treatment. Gary was using a stick to help him walk. He explained that he had injured his spine in a workplace accident some five years previously and was in constant pain.

His face was strained as he lay down on the treatment couch. As hands were placed on him, Gary began to relax. During his treatment, one or two other practitioners joined in.

At the end of the treatment, Gary was smiling broadly. He confided that for the first time since the accident he was pain-free. He cautiously stood up without the aid of his walking stick, amazed by what had happened.

Gary hadn't been interested in experiencing Reiki. It was his wife, Ros, who had persuaded him. Being sceptical, he'd doubted it could help.

Gary and Ros decided to learn Reiki. Before training, Gary had been taking painkillers continually. Since then, he hasn't needed to. Gary has managed the pain using Reiki. He is so pleased to have found a therapy that not only helps him but is also something he can do for himself.

HANNAH'S STORY

One of the satellite television channels invited us to talk about Reiki on one of their live, afternoon shows. During the interview, viewers were invited to call in. A woman we'll call Hannah phoned in, wanting to share what turned out to be a fascinating story.

Her husband had been diagnosed with an inoperable brain tumour and his outlook was poor. He was offered Reiki to see if it could help. He decided to accept.

After several treatments, he returned to the hospital for a brain scan. While studying the results, the doctor was astonished to discover that the tumour had moved.

He couldn't explain why, but said that it was now in a place where it could be operated upon. Despite the risk involved, the woman's husband went ahead with the operation. Her voice became emotional as she described the joy she felt when he made a full recovery.

PAULA'S MIRACLE

Paula had a hole-in-the-heart condition and accepted she would have to endure a number of symptoms all her life. One day she agreed to have a Reiki treatment, although she didn't have a clear idea of what it was. Paula didn't mention her condition, as she didn't feel it was relevant. She was stressed and over-tired. Paula hoped this treatment might help, but had no idea what was to come.

During the treatment, she was aware of something unusual happening. Having never experienced Reiki, she thought it was either something that occurred on a regular basis, or was simply her imagination playing tricks.

When the treatment ended, she felt energized and relaxed. She was taken aback when the practitioner then asked whether she had any kind of problem in her heart area. When she told him about the condition, he went on to tell her that it had been healed.

Having no idea whether or not this could be true, Paula didn't know what to say. She thanked him and went on her way. Some time later, she returned to the doctor for routine tests. To her astonishment, she was told that, inexplicably, the hole in the heart had healed.

Our hearts have been touched on many occasions by the incredible events we have been privileged to witness. While we never hold a particular expectation in mind, it is always special when change occurs, especially when it makes a significant difference to the quality of a person's life.

A FULL TREATMENT

Demonstrations are a great way to experience Reiki, and while short hands-on treatments are helpful, a full treatment is ideal. This takes about an hour. It is usual to lie down, ideally on a treatment table, covered by a light blanket if it is cool. Other than taking off an outdoor coat and shoes, you would be fully clothed for the treatment.

The practitioner usually explains what happens during a treatment, so you have an idea of what to expect. Sometimes, relaxing music is played. Some practitioners place essential oils in a burner to give off a pleasant aroma. Whatever the setting, the environment is conducive to relaxation, letting you make the most of the experience.

During the session, hands are placed in a number of positions on both the front and back of the body. If a person expresses the need for attention to be given to a particular area, then it is likely this part will be focused upon. However, this is not always the case, as Reiki tends to treat the underlying causes of dis-ease, rather than focusing on individual symptoms. The practitioner may start to treat a particular area, only to find another area is drawing a lot more energy. When this happens, the practitioner follows his or her instincts.

Everyone experiences Reiki differently. Some fall asleep immediately and are unaware of anything for the duration. Others feel tingling, vibration or warmth. Sometimes tears surface. Usually people experience a blissful, euphoric feeling, which they find soothing.

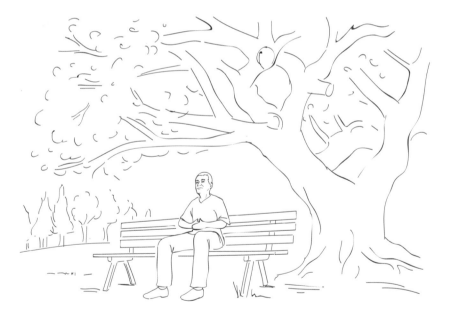

FITTING REIKI INTO A BUSY DAY

Reiki can be fitted into the busiest of days, being the perfect antidote to stress. It is an invaluable tool for restoring depleted energy. Those who have taken Reiki training use it anywhere, because all you need are your hands.

It is possible to use Reiki to rebalance the system before an illness manifests. The benefits of calming the mind down at an early stage cannot be over-stated. Clear thinking can go a long way towards the prevention of possible accidents, whether in the home, workplace or while driving. If a short treatment isn't possible and you succumb to a headache or an infection, then Reiki can help minimize the symptoms and bring early relief.

It is easy to give yourself a quick treatment during a busy day. Whether travelling, sitting at a desk, waiting for an appointment, while the children are out or while the baby is sleeping, there is usually some opportunity. Even if you are not alone, it is possible to place your hands discreetly on your stomach area, without anyone being aware that you are letting the energy flow through your system.

For further details on using Reiki with specific conditions and symptoms, see Part II.

6 How Reiki Works

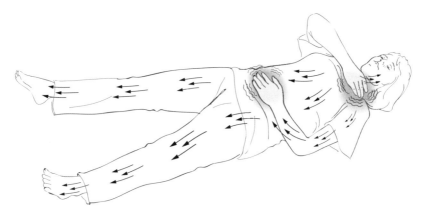

THE ATTUNEMENT PROCESS

'Attunements' are at the core of the Usui system of healing, and are the key to Reiki. They are also one of the main differences between Reiki and other healing modalities, being the catalyst for the amplification of life-force energy.

For students of Reiki, the initiation process aligns the system energetically, creating a new pathway through which energy can flow. The procedure involves using a precise technique combining symbols and mantras in a way that allows the creation of a strengthened connection between the person and universal life-force energy. A number of these attunements take place during Reiki classes.

In order to gain a pure and complete connection to Reiki energy, it is important to be attuned by a qualified Reiki teacher. It is not enough to have read a book or practised some techniques. The attunements are a physical and energetic transmission from teacher to student. Not all forms of Reiki are the same. Its oral tradition and growing popularity has meant that some material has been altered over time. Some Reiki masters have added or removed parts, making it their own. It is essential to be attuned by a teacher who has received the teachings and energetically integrated the wisdom through a direct connection with a living master.

THE CAUSE OF ILLNESS

There are many reasons why illness is caused. In addition to factors such as heredity, environment, nutrition and level of physical activity, the emotions and thoughts affect the body, helping to mould its very fabric.

The brain can be likened to a super-computer registering and retaining thoughts. The mind functions through the etheric body, leaving an impression on the physical. Whereas positive energy keeps the body supple and flexible, negative energy creates blocks and restrictions in the etheric, causing the physical body to stiffen up. Massage therapists experience this daily as tightness in their clients' muscles.

Whenever we have a strong, emotional reaction to an event, our thoughts and feelings around it become stored in the cellular structure of the body. Fear, anger and grief cause the muscles to assume certain positions and can lead to rigidity. If issues are not dealt with or released, a person's life-force energy can become restricted or even blocked.

Reiki is a simple and effective way to heal emotional blocks and restore inner balance. A person's awareness is raised by the heightened energy flow. The process highlights unhelpful thought patterns, often facilitating their release. Emotional blockages dissolve, relieving physical symptoms and enabling healing to occur.

Before a treatment, we always suggest a person decides where he or she would like the energy to go in life. There is no need to say this aloud. Alternatively, the person can ask a question such as 'What is the most important direction for me to take right now?' Answers can be enlightening and revealing.

Kay was a person always keen to help. She was generous with her time and had lots of energy. Kay became so used to helping, assisting and volunteering her time that, as she got older, it became more and more difficult for her to say no.

One day, she was diagnosed with lymphoma. Following chemotherapy, her energy was low. She struggled to live her life at the usual pace. Kay (reluctantly) allowed others to help her, and we were privileged to give her some Reiki. After one treatment, she shared an important insight. Kay had asked why she had developed cancer. During the treatment, she had the answer: The illness was saying 'no' for her. She was shocked to realize this may have contributed to her condition.

Louise Hay, in her book *You Can Heal Your Life*, suggests that many physical illnesses originate in the mind. It is her belief that if the thought-processes that created the illness were cleared, there would be a good chance it would not reoccur.

As a five-year-old child, Louise Hay was raped and battered. Later she developed vaginal cancer. As a teacher and adult, she realized this was no coincidence. Cutting the cancer away may not be enough, she realized, if she continued to carry the pattern of deep resentment around what happened to her.

Louise Hay worked intensively on herself for six months, cleansing and strengthening her body through nutrition and exercise. She worked hard to deal with the pain and resentment of her inner suffering. Louise managed to heal herself. Her story, and her subsequent books, became an inspiration to millions.

In *Heal Your Body*, Louise lists possible mental patterns behind many physical illnesses, compiled from her years of experience with her clients. While metaphysical causations are not definitive, it is always worth considering whether they have contributed to a dis-ease state. For this reason, we include some emotional causes for physical illnesses in Part II.

7 Self-treatment

There are a number of hand positions which are a useful guide to self-treatment (see Chapter 9). They can be easily adapted for effective 15-minute sessions as referred to in Part II. If you haven't yet taken Reiki training, you can still benefit, as we all have energy flowing through our systems. Reiki training enhances that energetic connection, allowing you to benefit more fully.

CREATE YOUR OWN SANCTUARY

Tension is who you think you should be.
Relaxation is who you are.
CHINESE PROVERB

Create a special place in your home where you can relax on your own. Choose somewhere away from the bustle of a busy household. An ideal place could be a sunlit window seat or a favourite armchair piled up with cushions. It could be a garden shed converted into your sanctuary. Or simply your bedroom, where you can shut the door on the world for a few moments.

Let yourself be creative. Set the scene for the kind of environment that could work for you. Soften the lighting, play evocative music or burn scented candles. Cushions or a favourite throw can add an inviting element.

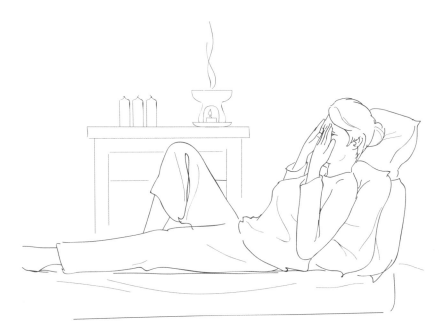

GIVING YOURSELF A TREATMENT

Having created some space, make yourself comfortable, either sitting or lying down. When placing your hands it is best if they are slightly cupped with your fingers together. Practice will determine whether a touch is too heavy or too light.

Aim to stay in each Position for 5 minutes. To gauge the time successfully it can be helpful to play music with timed intervals. There are many such albums available. However, the time spent at each Position is not critical and does not need to be timed. It is just a guide. Guessing the time or allowing yourself to be guided by your intuition can be equally effective. Students have told us of instances when they've left their hands too long in a Position, only to find it was just what was required.

A treatment can take up to an hour. It's a great way to increase strength and improve well-being in addition to recharging your batteries.

FINDING TIME FOR YOURSELF

In our fast-paced lives there often isn't time for a full treatment, so choose to treat the areas most needing energy. The following is included as a general guideline.

When there is only time for three 5-minute Positions, a suggestion is to place your hands over your eyes (Position 1), over your heart (Position 5) and over your abdomen (Position 7).

Be resourceful. Perhaps you can make the most of a brief period while the baby sleeps or, if you are a home-worker, plan to put the answering machine on while you disappear to a quiet room for 15 minutes. If you can't do this because your workplace is outside the home, find a quiet park bench during a lunch or coffee break, or some indoor space where you are unlikely to be disturbed. If you have your own office, divert all calls and put a notice on the door.

It may be difficult for a student to find time, so plan ahead. Early morning might be a good time, before others are up or after they have left to attend lectures. Giving others advanced warning and putting a reminder on the door may help.

Travelling is often prolonged and stressful. It can offer opportunities to discreetly give yourself some Reiki. You can do this whether sitting in a waiting room, on an aircraft, or in a car, train or bus.

The early part of a holiday is often spent recuperating from the journey. Having arrived, treating yourself outdoors in a natural environment is one of the best ways of receiving Reiki. Whether it's on a beach, by a lake or in the mountains, a treatment outside is blissfully relaxing and restorative.

8 Treating Others

*Often we underestimate the power of a touch, a smile, a kind
word, a listening ear, an honest compliment, or the smallest act
of caring, all of which have the potential to turn a life around.*
LEO BUSCAGLIA

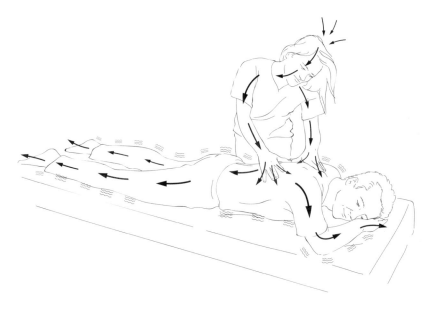

When giving a treatment, make sure the person is comfortable before you
begin. Explain about the hand positions. Treatments can be given to a person who is either sitting or lying down. Full treatments last about an hour,
using 12 basic hand Positions – or more depending on the circumstances.
Except for after a particular shock or accident, give Reiki to the entire body
whenever possible.

Short treatments may be appropriate if a person is in pain or cannot remain still for long. Young children tend to let you know when they have had enough!

In certain circumstances it is not appropriate to give Reiki. For example, following a pre-operative anaesthetic. Reiki increases awareness, which might not be helpful. Reiki would, however, speed up healing after an operation.

If for any reason a person feels uncomfortable during a Reiki treatment, it is best to discontinue. Usually a person will tell you, or it may become apparent by their body language.

SCANNING TECHNIQUE

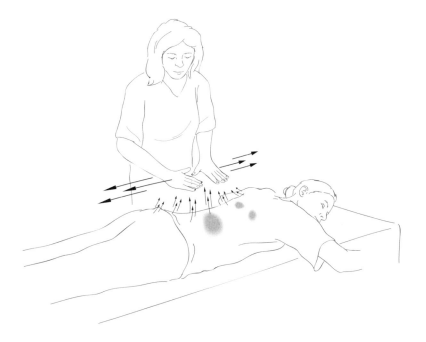

Scanning a person's body before a treatment can help determine where energy is most needed.

To begin, stand alongside the person. With your hands 5 or 6 centimetres above the body, move slowly along the length of the body, from head to foot. Notice any areas that feel especially warm or particularly cool. Be aware of the sensation in your hands. Concentrate on your hands' experience as they move over the body. Do they feel tingly or prickly in a particular area?

While scanning, you are working in the person's energetic field or aura, where it is possible to sense imbalances before they manifest physically. Through this simple technique you can detect where energy is needed. Usually, more energy is required in areas where your hands encounter a subtle difference in body temperature.

GUIDE TO INTERPRETING IMPRESSIONS

Heat

Indicates energy is needed. Spend more time on this area. Usually this heat dissipates during the treatment.

Coolness

This could be an emotional or spiritual energetic block. It may indicate repressed feelings and require repeated treatments to clear. If the area proves resistant, bodywork such as Rolfing may help to release deep-seated feelings.

Visual Impressions

Assist the understanding of the person's condition and may be communicated to them, if appropriate.

Dull Pain

Could imply a physical problem or damage from the past, such as scar tissue.

Hands feel drawn to an Area

Sometimes the hands feel almost magnetically drawn to an area. This indicates an area of the body in particular need.

Hands feel repelled from an Area

This feeling of being repelled from a part of the body can indicate deep-seated issues the person is reluctant to face. Ascertain whether the person is ready to deal with these blockages before giving this area more energy.

Sharp Pain

This indicates a build-up of energy in the area. It could be due to a recent physical problem. Reiki will help to accelerate the healing process.

Tingling

Tingling can indicate inflammation. If there is no obvious cause it may be there is suppressed anger, not acknowledged at a conscious level. The knees and jaw often store much anger. Reiki can help feelings come to the surface so the person can deal with them and move on.

Vibration

Can indicate a chakra imbalance. Sometimes the person receiving the treatment feels a subtle vibration, while you do not. Everyone processes an experience differently. Usually the chakra concerned becomes rebalanced during the treatment.

SWEEPING TECHNIQUE

Following the treatment, sweep down the etheric field to clear energetic debris released during the treatment. Working from head to toe, place the hands 6 or 7 centimetres above the body. In a sideways motion, sweep across the energetic field from head to toe and just beyond. Imagine any energy disposed of being absorbed into the earth or melting away into the ether.

THE DIVERSITY OF REIKI

Reiki can successfully treat children of all ages, as well as animals, plants and even trees. Some practitioners train in order to use Reiki specifically with horses. We've heard some remarkable stories illustrating how helpful Reiki has been with animals, and are always amazed to hear how resourceful people are.

Monty's Cough

As a Reiki Master, Doreen had treated many people, but had never given Reiki to an animal. One Sunday morning she was driving along a country lane when she saw her friend Cath standing by the roadside with her horse, Monty. Monty had become distressed by a severe cough. Cath explained that the bouts of coughing had brought him down onto his front knees, and that they were awaiting help.

Cath asked Doreen whether she could give Monty some Reiki. Monty was a large horse, aged about 12. With some difficulty, Doreen managed to place her hands on Monty's spine and heart. After about 15 minutes he moved away, indicating he had received enough energy. Doreen stopped treating him and continued on her way. About an hour later, on her return, Doreen saw Cath and Monty still waiting on the roadside. Doreen again treated Monty and then returned home.

Next day, Doreen received an excited call from Cath. Monty's cough had disappeared and he did not need the prescribed medication.

Penelope's Travel Sickness

A friend of ours, Jeremy, told us that his daughter Penelope suffered from travel sickness. He joked that she became ill even when driving her own car. When she won a trip to Australia, the thought of the 24-hour flight made the journey seem more of an ordeal than a glittering prize. Jeremy sent distant healing to Penelope, using a procedure learned at Second Degree level. To his astonishment she reported suffering no travel sickness on the journey, nor on any of the other flights she took while in Australia. Her enjoyment of the trip was complete.

THE SIMPLICITY OF REIKI

The applications of Reiki are extensive and limited only by the imagination. Ailing plants can be revived, family pets helped, and babies treated before and after birth. Reiki can be used to calm a person down or energize someone who is flagging. It can boost confidence and revitalize. It can even be sent to someone far away.

Reiki is the most simple, therapeutic form of healing we know. It is easily learned and straightforward to use. In the next Part we suggest how you can treat everyday symptoms and chronic conditions with Reiki, however much time you have available.

9 Hand Positions for Reiki Treatments

Before starting a treatment, it is particularly calming to place hands briefly on the shoulders, as shown.

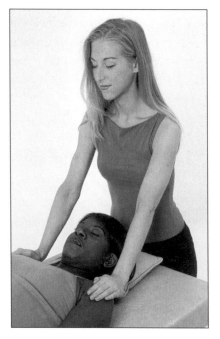

Pre-treatment position

Position 1

Over the forehead, eyes and cheeks. Helps relieve stress, headaches and cold symptoms. Improves clarity and concentration, and enhances focus and decision-making.

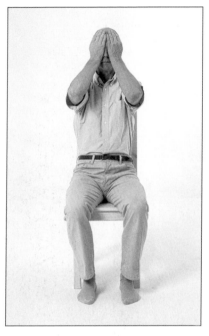
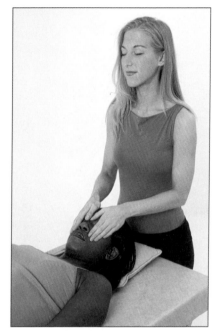

Position 1 (self)   Position 1 (others)

Position 2

The temples. Helps to relieve headaches and migraines. Soothes shock. Assists the release of worry, stress and depression. Creativity is enhanced. Memory and dream-recall improve.

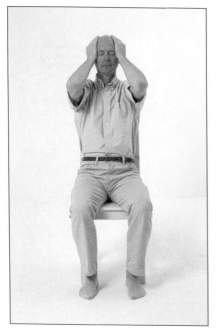

Position 2 (self)

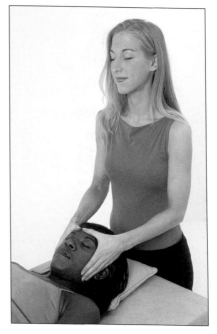

Position 2 (others)

Position 3

Back of the head. This releases stress, anxiety and depression. Calms the mind. Helpful for pain-relief, nausea and for raising self-esteem. Assists headaches, migraines and head injuries.

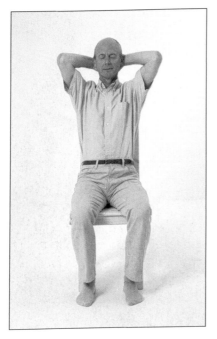

Position 3 (self)

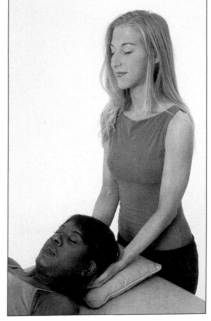

Position 3 (others)

Position 4

Over the throat and along the jaw line. Stimulates and treats metabolic disorders. Relieves sore throats, swollen glands and symptoms of the flu. Helps improve weight problems. Addresses anger, hostility and resentment. Improves confidence, joy, communication and self-expression.

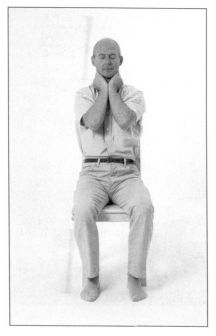

Position 4 (self)

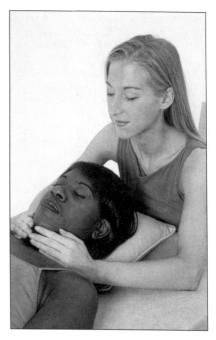

Position 4 (others)

Position 5

Over the heart. Releases pent-up emotions and stress. Treats heart palpitations and angina. Restores balance and harmony. Releases fear. Improves blood circulation. Enhances the capacity to love and be loved.

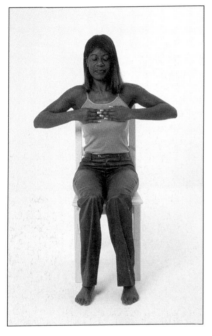

Position 5 (self)

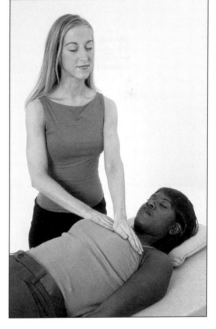

Position 5 (others)

Position 6

Over the solar plexus area, just below the chest. Improves confidence, security, inner power and relaxation. Releases anxiety and apprehension. Brings clarity to the decision-making process.

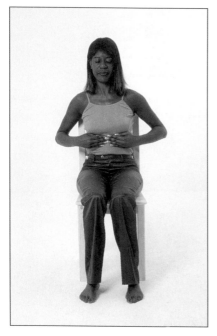

Position 6 (self)

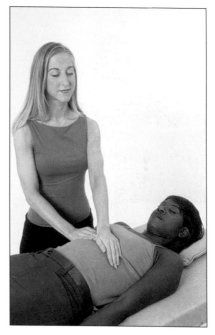

Position 6 (others)

Position 7

Over the abdomen. This calms the emotions. It assists the release of anger, resentment, bitterness and frustration. Restores inner balance and harmony.

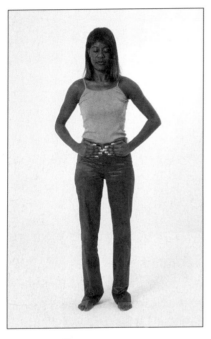

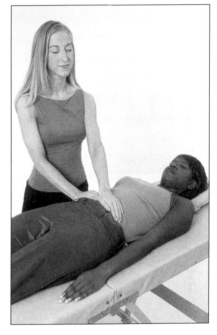

Position 7 (self)

Position 7 (others)

Position 8

Over the pelvic area. Helps speed up the release of toxins. Releases emotions such as frustration, guilt and feelings of insecurity. Improves confidence and creativity. Brings balance to sexual issues. For women, relieves menstrual symptoms and prevents ovarian cysts. For men, helps prevent prostate problems.

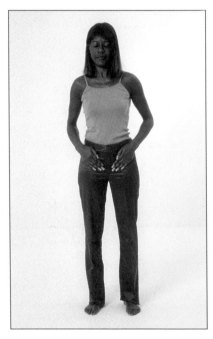

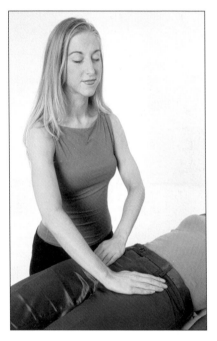

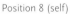
Position 8 (self)

Position 8 (others)

Position 9

Over the knees. Relieves resentment, insecurity and fear of change. Releases anger and improves emotional balance.

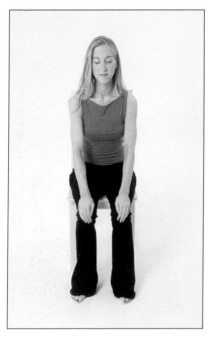

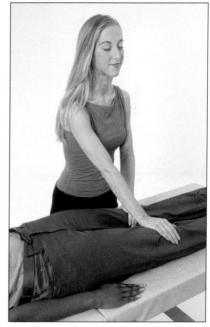

Position 9 (self)

Position 9 (others)

Position 10

Over the feet. Is grounding, soothing and nurturing.

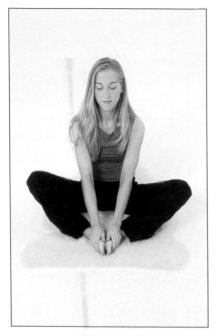

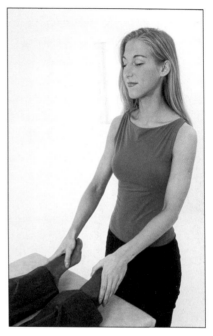

Position 10 (self)

Position 10 (others)

Position 11

Self-treatment at the base of the neck. Relieves muscle tension and neck problems. Assists in preventing migraines. Enhances the ability to love and be loved. Releases feelings of self-doubt and worry.

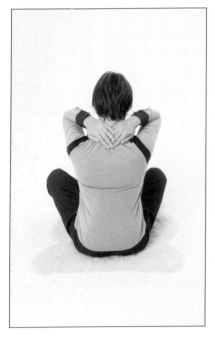

Position 11 (self)

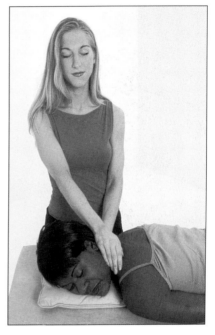

Position 11 (others)

Position 12

Over the top of the shoulders. Releases tension stored in the shoulder area. Brings harmony and relief from stress.

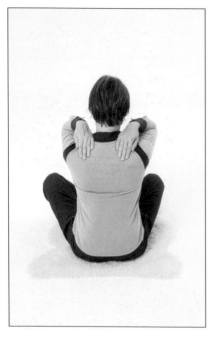

Position 12 (self)

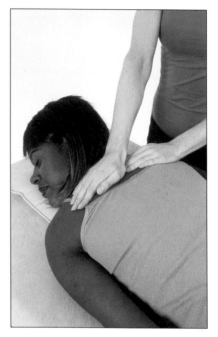

Position 12 (others)

Position 13

When treating another this is over the back of the heart. Improves emotional balance. Helps love to flow through the heart.

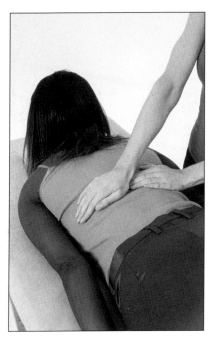

Position 13 (others)

Position 14

Around the waist and lower back. Releases feelings of self-criticism and anxiety. Allows difficult situations to be viewed in a more positive way.

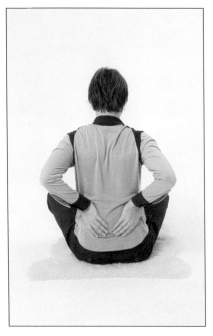

Position 14 (self)

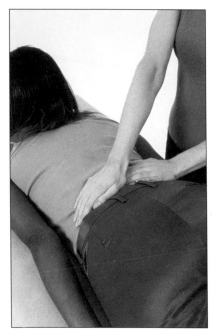

Position 14 (others)

Position 15

Over the base of the spine. Excellent for stress-release, backache, sciatica and hip problems. Helps with creativity and innovation. Lets go old feelings and thoughts, making room for new, creative expression and innovation.

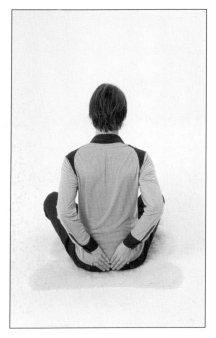
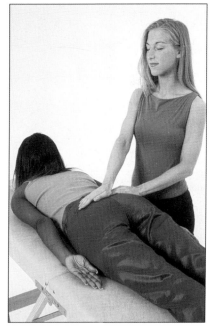

Position 15 (self)   Position 15 (others)

Position 16

Over the soles of the feet. As the reflex points are located in the feet, treating this area gives an energetic boost to the whole body.

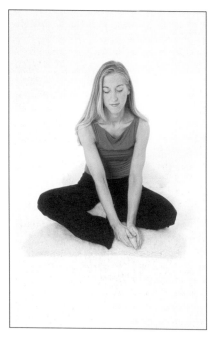 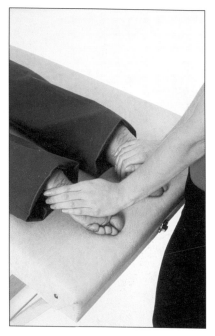

Position 16 (self)

Position 16 (others)

When treating others, bring the treatment to a close by placing one hand on the base of the spine and the other at the top of the head for a couple of minutes. This has a helpful, grounding effect on the person being treated.

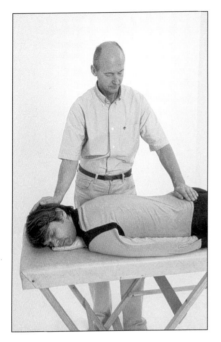

ending a treatment

PART TWO

10 Everyday Complaints

While full-body treatments are ideal, some positions are particularly help-ful with certain conditions or symptoms.

The hand positions referred to in this chapter are illustrated in Chapter 9.

Back Pain

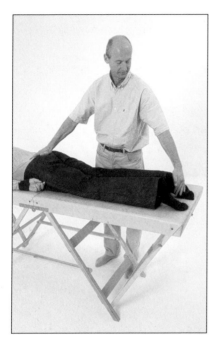

15-MINUTE TREATMENT

Treat directly over the area of discomfort. For a short treatment, place one hand on the base of the spine and the other on the sole of one foot. After 5 minutes, change to the other foot.

If you have time for a longer treatment, use the positions that directly treat the back area from the shoulders down to the base of the spine (Positions 12 to 15). It is also helpful to take the energy right down to the feet (Position 16).

Possible Causes

Pain in the upper back can be caused by lack of emotional support, feeling unloved and isolated. Can also result from holding back love, or becoming overwhelmed by too much responsibility.

Pain the middle back may be a result of guilt or remorse for something that happened in the past.

Pain in the lower back could be due to lack of financial support and feelings of pressure in times of uncertainty. Having to put on a brave face when confronted with difficulty or lack of abundance. Could also relate to matters of a sexual nature.

Other Suggestions

Stress has a lot to do with back pain, in addition to other factors. Avoid excess stress and take regular exercise. Aim to identify the source of muscle tension. If a physical one, such as sitting for lengthy periods, make changes to your routine. Notice if a particular emotion (such as anger, for example) leads to back pain. Don't let yourself hold on to it.

Yoga can help keep the spine and its surrounding muscles supple. There are different types of yoga to suit different people. A lesser-known form, called viniyoga, emphasizes the importance of using a personalized programme that takes back injuries into account. One-to-one lessons with a viniyoga practitioner can produce such a plan (see viniyoga website address on page 197).

Turmeric is recommended by ayurvedic practitioners to relieve painful injuries.

Colds and Flu

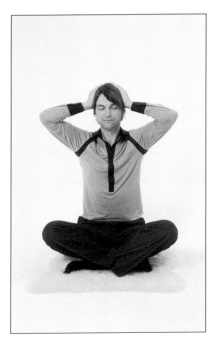

15-MINUTE TREATMENT

Place the hands over the eyes for 5 minutes (Position 1) then above the ears followed by the sides and front of the throat (Position 4).

Possible Causes

Colds are usually caused by lack of space and having too much to do. It's also a sign of needing time to integrate life experiences and deal with emotional issues.

Other Suggestions

Drink plenty of fluids and enjoy the space. We find that taking 250 mg echinacea three times a day, 1,000 mg vitamin C every few hours, 2 x 25 mg zinc after each meal and 300 mg elderberry extract three times a day in addition to Reiki stops a cold in its tracks.

If the cold does invade the system, inhalations of lavender, tea tree, eucalyptus, peppermint and rosemary all help clear the nasal passages.

Constipation

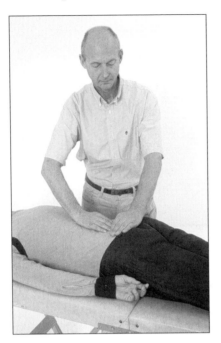

15-MINUTE TREATMENT

Place the hands over the abdomen area in Position 7. Place one hand over the lower back and the other over the base of the spine, forming a T-shape with your hands.

Possible Causes

This condition is sometimes caused by resistance to releasing old ideas. It can be a case of being stuck in the past.

Other Suggestions

Drink lots of water, take a brisk walk daily and make sure your diet contains plenty of green leafy vegetables, fruit and whole grains. Don't hold on to any old thought-patterns that don't serve you any longer and go with the flow.

Coughs

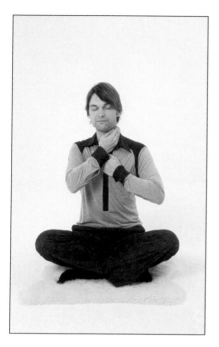

15-MINUTE TREATMENT

Place the hands along the jaw line (Position 4) for 5 minutes, then place your hands a little lower, one hand across the top of the chest and the other across the base of the throat area for another 5 minutes. If more time is available, treat the upper back as well.

Possible Causes

A cough can be indicative of needing to get something off your chest. Ask yourself what it is you need to say to someone.

Other Suggestions

There are excellent homoeopathic remedies for coughs, depending on the symptoms. Aconite helps a hard, barking cough. Dr Usui used to suggest a hot drink made from grated ginger and honey. Rubbing the chest with tiger balm can help.

Cystitis

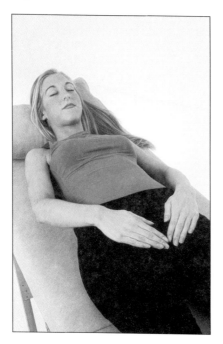

15-MINUTE TREATMENT

Treat the genital area directly, as shown. Then place your hands over the pelvic region (Position 8) for a further 5 minutes. When treating others, it is not appropriate to treat the genital area directly.

Possible Causes

This infection can result from an impaired immune system. At an emotional level, cystitis could be caused by anxiety and a fear of letting go.

Other Suggestions

Eat wholegrain foods and plenty of organic fruit, vegetables and salads to build up your immune system. Drink cranberry juice, kombucha tea and plenty of water each day. Affirm that you easily and comfortably let go of unwanted emotions and welcome new opportunities into your life.

Diarrhoea

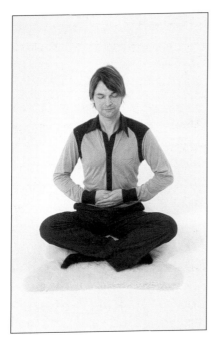

15-MINUTE TREATMENT

Place one hand on top of the other over the stomach. If more time is available, place your hands on the abdomen and then on to the pelvic area (Positions 6 to 8). Also, treat the lower back and base of the spine (Positions 14 and 15).

Possible Causes

Can be caused by bacteria or parasitic infections as well as poisoning. Can also be created by psychological problems. This condition is often fear-based. It can be brought on by a refusal to be open to new ideas, rejecting concepts without considering new possibilities.

Other Suggestions

Take probiotics before travelling to strengthen the immune system and protect against parasitic infections. Recommended are FOS supplements and acidophilus, both of which are available from health food shops.

For everyday prevention of this condition, avoid any foods you find difficult to digest. Drink plenty of fluids. At an emotional level, aim to slow down and take time to consider options more carefully. Don't let fear cloud your judgement. Make decisions calmly. Keep a journal, so you can write out anything that is bothering you.

Ear Infections

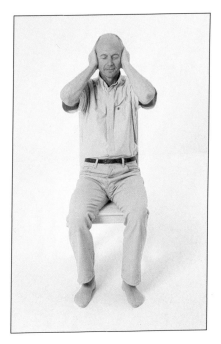

15-MINUTE TREATMENT

Place your hands directly over the ears for several minutes. Then move to Position 4 along the jaw line and throat area.

Possible Causes

Feeling out of sorts. Too much external turmoil you don't want to hear.

Other Suggestions

Tea tree oil or tiger balm can be helpful, massaged onto the outer ear and neck region. Remove yourself from inharmonious atmospheres and find peace in a tranquil environment. Send out loving thoughts to others and to any situation you find difficult. Give yourself Reiki as described above and allow yourself to return to a position of balance.

Fever

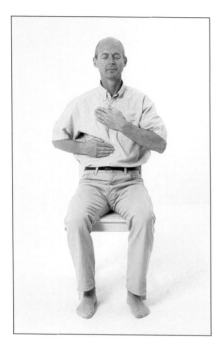

15-MINUTE TREATMENT

Treat the solar plexus, abdomen and pelvic area (Positions 6 to 8) to encourage the toxin-eliminating organs. Place one hand across the chest and the other over the liver, above and to the right of the abdomen area.

Possible Causes

A fever is the body's way of fighting an infection. At an emotional level, it can be caused by anger and inner conflict.

Other Suggestions

Eat lightly and drink plenty of fluids. Calm the mind and rest as much as possible.

Flatulence

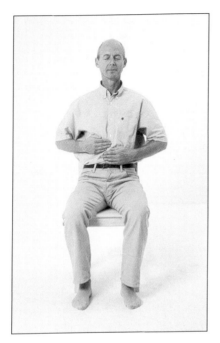

15-MINUTE TREATMENT

Treat the abdomen and pelvic area (Positions 7 and 8). Also, treat the digestive area by placing hands over the liver and spleen, as shown in the photograph.

Possible Causes

This condition can be caused by undigested feelings and fear-based reactions to new ideas.

Other Suggestions

Eat slowly, ensuring you combine foods carefully. Take time to digest new ideas and concepts. Meditation is recommended to still the mind and increase clarity.

Food Intolerances

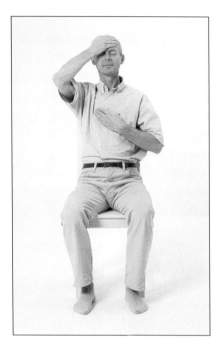

15-MINUTE TREATMENT

Place one hand on the forehead and the other over the heart. Treat the eyes, the back of the head, the solar plexus and abdomen (Positions 1, 3, 6 and 7).

Possible Causes

Food intolerances indicate that the body has become stressed. The intolerance may be a perfectly appropriate response to a substance the body cannot tolerate. Alternatively, it can result from the body over-reacting to an otherwise harmless substance. At an emotional level, can indicate unwillingness to integrate aspects of your personality that you are not comfortable with.

Other Suggestions

Ensure you are eating the food your body can digest. Identify the foods that are affecting you. Keeping a food diary is one of the easiest ways. Record every food you eat and note when you have an adverse reaction. Eliminate suspect foods. Many people find they cannot tolerate foods that contain dairy products or wheat.

A cleansing diet under the supervision of a nutritionist can restore balance. Build up your immune system with 1,000 mg vitamin C daily, plus zinc, cat's claw and echinacea. Switch to organic fruit and vegetables. Read Peter D'Adamo's 'Eat Right For Your Type' to ensure your diet is compatible with your blood type.

To prevent further problems, take the supplement quercetin, which is a natural product. It stabilizes the membranes of cells that release histamine and helps many allergic responses.

Affirm unconditional self-love. If you feel you have issues preventing you accepting yourself for all that you are, you may choose to work with the support of a therapist.

Fungal Infections

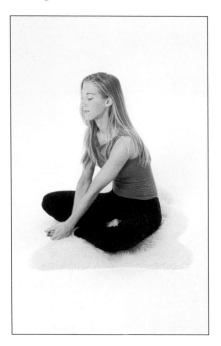

15-MINUTE TREATMENT

Treat the solar plexus, stomach and pelvic area (Positions 6 to 8). Place one hand under and one over the foot (or the area needing treatment) to encase the area. Change feet.

Possible Causes

Fungal infections such as athlete's foot can sometimes indicate a frustration at not being accepted. It can suggest a reluctance to move forwards.

Other Suggestions

Herbal tinctures can help to cleanse the system. Eat plenty of leafy green vegetables to strengthen the immune system. A detoxification diet can help rid the body of stored toxins.

Decide here and now to love and approve of yourself. If any self-critical thoughts arise, simply say 'cancel, cancel' to yourself and let them go.

Haemorrhoids

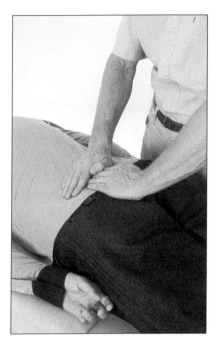

15-MINUTE TREATMENT

Treat the abdomen area (Position 7) and the base of the spine (Position 15). Place one hand across the base of the spine and the other across the lower spine, forming a T-shape.

Possible Causes

This condition can be created by feeling burdened either by a present situation or by what has happened in the past. It suggests that there is resistance to letting go.

Other Suggestions

Allow yourself to feel that there is the time and space for everything you want to do. Move forward with confidence, knowing that you can release anything that has been holding you back. Take regular exercise. Eat a nutritious diet that is high in fibre. Include fresh garlic in your diet and drink kombucha. (Details on kombucha can be found on page 196.)

Headaches

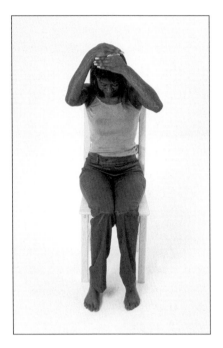

15-MINUTE TREATMENT

Dr Usui recommended placing your hands on the head until the pain has gone. Treat the headache using the head positions, especially over the temples. Another position across the top of the head can be helpful.

Possible Causes

Headaches are often caused by dehydration. Ensure you have plenty of water to drink throughout the day. Inner conflict can also create a headache, as can forcing an overtired mind to continue when it wants a break.

Other Suggestions

During busy days, give yourself an adequate number of breaks. Don't let yourself work under excessive pressure. Allow enough time to make difficult decisions. Meditation is a helpful way to calm the mind. Indian head massage is excellent for releasing tension.

Indigestion

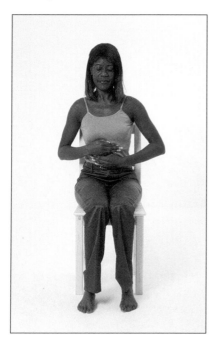

15-MINUTE TREATMENT

Treat the solar plexus, abdomen and pelvic area (Positions 6 to 8). Place both hands next to each other over the pancreas under the chest as shown.

Possible Causes

Indigestion can be caused by feelings of anxiety. Worry and concern over loss of control in your life can contribute, as can apprehension. Fear is often internalized in the gut area and can cause considerable discomfort.

Other Suggestions

Relax and trust that everything will work out in the most appropriate way. Acknowledge your feelings and choose to harness your inner power so that you can comfortably deal with challenges that come your way.

Insomnia

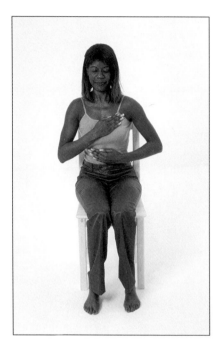

15-MINUTE TREATMENT

Reiki is excellent for insomnia as it quickly induces a state of deep relaxation. Treat the eyes (Position 1) and use the other head positions (Positions 2, 3 and 4). Also, place one hand on the solar plexus and the other across the heart (Positions 5 and 6).

Possible Causes

There can be many causes for insomnia including anxiety, depression, drinking stimulants such as coffee or excess environmental noise. It is also caused by feelings of vulnerability and a refusal to trust in a positive outcome.

Other Suggestions

Give yourself a Reiki treatment before going to sleep, or meditate, focusing on your breathing. You may want to write in your journal before going to sleep. Committing your thoughts to paper can release them from the mind. At a practical level, avoid caffeine and other stimulants in the latter part of the day. Homoeopathic remedies are helpful for insomnia, as is hypnotherapy. To calm and still the mind, allow yourself to trust that you are safe and let your intuition guide you.

Suggest to yourself that whenever your hands are placed over your eyes, you will immediately sink into a deep state of relaxation.

Itching

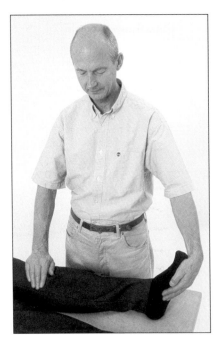

15-MINUTE TREATMENT

Place your hands over the solar plexus and abdomen areas (Positions 6 and 7), followed by the shoulder blades and lower back (Positions 13 and 14). Also, place one hand on the knee and the other on the sole of the foot. Change feet.

Possible Causes

Itching usually suggests that someone or something is irritating. Take a moment to consider who or what is causing you to feel so sensitive. Are you itching to be elsewhere?

Other Suggestions

A detoxification diet will help desensitize the system. Fasting for a couple of days on plenty of juices made from fresh vegetables, plus hot vegetable broths, can transform your system. Dry skin brushing before a shower is helpful. Relax, go with the flow and know that all your needs will be met.

Jet Lag

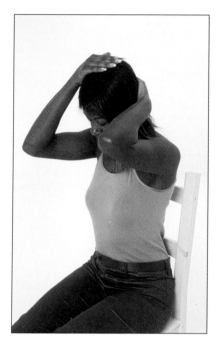

15-MINUTE TREATMENT

Place your hands over the eyes, then over the temples (Positions 1 and 2), followed by the solar plexus and abdomen (Positions 6 and 7). Place one hand on the crown of the head and the other on the back of the neck.

Possible Causes

Crossing time zones can disrupt sleep patterns, causing the body to feel extremely stressed. The aircraft's environment is lower in oxygen than we are used to, resulting in a dry onboard atmosphere.

Other Suggestions

Drink plenty of fluids, avoiding alcohol, tea and coffee, as they are too dehydrating. Take an anti-stress, time-release 1,000 mg of vitamin C and a high potency B-complex vitamin before the flight. The hormone melatonin can be helpful, but it must be taken at the bedtime of your destination to be effective, and continued for a few days after your arrival (only available on prescription in the UK or via the Internet at the time of writing). A pair of fabric eyeshades is helpful. After you land, continue to drink plenty of fluids and take some light exercise to assist the body's readjustment.

Knee Problems

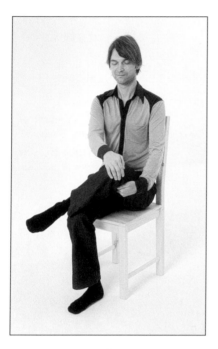

15-MINUTE TREATMENT

Treat the knee area directly (Position 9) plus the shoulder blades and lower back (Positions 13 and 14). This ensures that the kidneys are treated as well. Treat the arch of the knees.

Possible Causes

Some natural practitioners believe that knee problems relate to imbalances of energy in the kidneys. Anger is often stored in the knees. It can sometimes relate to inflexibility.

Other Suggestions

Strengthen the energy in the kidneys by taking Royal Jelly supplements. Release stress with meditation and visualization exercises. Take a walk or other light exercise to assist in the release of trapped energy. Embrace forgiveness so that you bend and flow with ease. Chinese medicine tinctures can also help. Consult a specialist practitioner (see page 196).

Leg Cramps

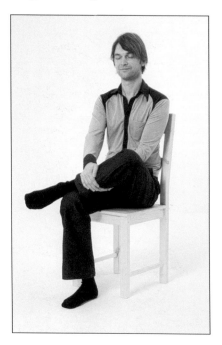

15-MINUTE TREATMENT

Treat the area directly as shown. Treat the knees and feet (Positions 9 and 10) as well as the kidneys and the area at the base of the spine (Positions 14 and 15). Place the hands on the tops of both shoulders.

Possible Causes

Cramps often indicate tension, fear and a resistance to move forwards. This can be due to a lack of emotional support while undergoing a period of confusion or change.

Other Suggestions

Relax and allow your mind to become calm and centred. Once you are peaceful, consider your options once again. Creative visualization can be helpful in making your decision.

Two cups of Epsom salts added to the bath can bring relief or you can make a massage oil from 6 drops each of clove and rosemary added to a carrier oil.

Mouth Ulcers

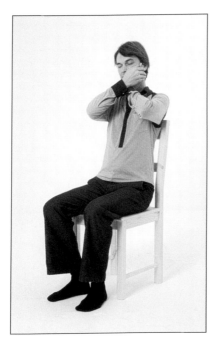

15-MINUTE TREATMENT

Place hands over either side of the mouth area to treat the ulcer directly. Treat the solar plexus, as well as the shoulder blades and lower back (Positions 6, 13 and 14).

Possible Causes

Cold sores are said to be a discharge of waste not cleansed by the liver and kidneys. This could indicate that the body's natural cleansing system is under par. On an emotional level this could be a negative response to a situation, or stem from withholding thoughts we are reluctant to express.

Other Suggestions

Detoxifying the system by fasting on carrot and apple juice for a day will help. Dab on a few drops of oil of St John's Wort. Ask yourself if you are uncomfortable with a situation.

Panic Attacks

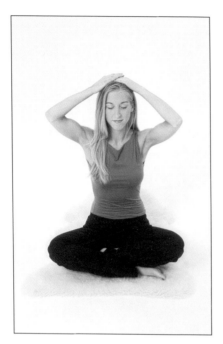

15-MINUTE TREATMENT

Treat the temples and back of the head (Positions 2 and 3) followed by the solar plexus and stomach (Positions 6 and 7). Finally, treat the crown chakra by placing both hands on top of the head.

Possible Causes

A panic attack occurs when feelings of anxiety become excessive. There are many causes. Generally they occur when a person feels unable to trust in the process of life and feels alone, vulnerable and unsupported. There is an overwhelming fear of loss of control over an outcome.

Other Suggestions

Hypnotherapy can be invaluable. You will learn useful relaxation techniques that can be used anywhere, and specific skills to deal with and overcome the attacks. Massage is beneficial. Avoid sugary foods and take regular exercise. A herbal supplement called *Relora* has been shown to reduce anxiety and increase feelings of relaxation. It works by reducing the levels of the stress hormones released when we feel anxious (www.relora.co.uk).

Let go of the need to control situations. Remember you are not alone, and ask for help at any time. Trust that everything will work out the way you want it to. Affirm that your needs will always be met and you are safe.

PMS (Pre-menstrual Syndrome)

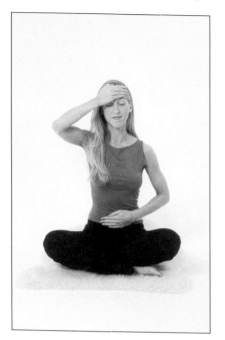

15-MINUTE TREATMENT

Treat the pelvic area and the base of the spine (Positions 8 and 15) as well as the heart area, if the breasts are tender (Position 5). Place one hand on the forehead and the other over the stomach area.

Possible Causes

Women often take on too much without taking the time to meet their own needs. Many put on a brave face and try to appear strong when they are feeling vulnerable.

Other Suggestions

Take regular supplements of evening primrose oil. Avoid excessive stress and eliminate caffeine from the diet. Eat plenty of organically-grown fruit and vegetables. Replace poly-unsaturated vegetable oils with extra-virgin cold-pressed olive oil. Use Reiki for relaxation and to relieve symptoms.

Sinusitis

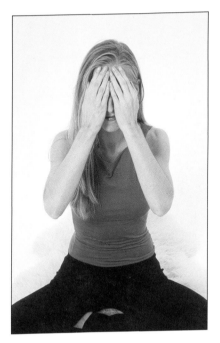

15-MINUTE TREATMENT

Place your hands over the eyes (Position 1) for at least 5 minutes. Then place the hands slightly lower down the face to treat the sinuses, as shown.

Possible Causes

Caused by infection in facial sinuses. At an emotional level, can be caused by being irritated by someone close to us or inability to express our feelings.

Other Suggestions

Dry skin brushing daily before a shower is helpful in stimulating draining of the sinuses. Bouncing on a mini-trampoline can be beneficial.

Relax and respond with love, affirming peace and harmony within yourself and surrounding you at all times. Traditional Chinese medicine can boost the immune system and relieve this condition.

Swollen Glands

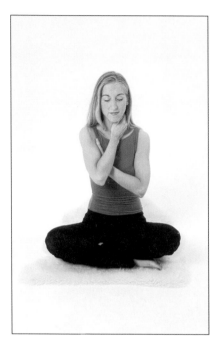

15-MINUTE TREATMENT

Place the hands alongside the jaw line over the throat (Position 4). Leave one hand over the throat and place the other in the armpit. Change.

Possible Causes

Swollen glands usually suggest the body is overloaded with toxins. It can also represent emotional issues that have not been dealt with. It indicates a weakened immune system.

Other Suggestions

Release yourself from inner conflict and be true to the person you are.

Dry skin brushing before a shower assists toxic elimination. Take a gentle walk each day. Eat plenty of leafy green vegetables and relax in a warm bath.

Tonsillitis

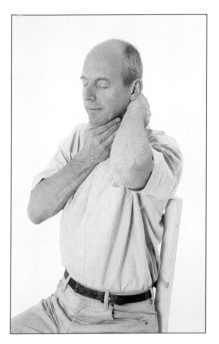

15-MINUTE TREATMENT

Treat along the jaw line over the throat (Position 4). Place one hand across the back of
the neck and the other across the throat area.

Possible Causes

Can indicate anger or fear surfacing. May be caused by being overwhelmed by a situation,
which is too much to swallow.

Other Suggestions

Rest and drink plenty of fluids. Release yourself from all restrictions. Avoid highly processed
foods and sweets. Include plenty of green vegetables and vegetable juices to detoxify the
system. Walking in natural surroundings can help to bring you back to harmony.

Toothache

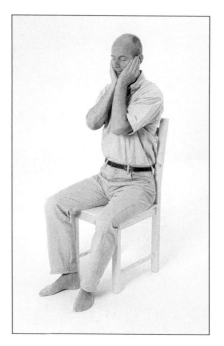

15-MINUTE TREATMENT

Treat the gums and teeth directly by placing your hands on either side of the mouth. Also, place hands across the jaw line (Position 4).

Possible Causes

This can be caused by a diet high in fat and sugar with too little fibrous content. At an emotional level, can indicate indecisiveness and uncertainty.

Other Suggestions

Go within and access your wisdom and intuition. Is there a decision you need to make or a direction you feel drawn to? Switch to a high quality diet to nourish and strengthen your system. Eat plenty of organic vegetables and fruit. Avoid sugar and refined foods.

Viral Infections

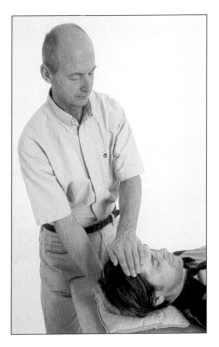

15-MINUTE TREATMENT

Place your hands over the eyes, temples, back of head and jaw line (Positions 1, 2, 3 and 4). Additionally, treat the chest, the abdomen, the shoulder blades and lower back (Positions 5, 7, 13 and 14). To treat others, place one hand on the back of the head and the other on the forehead.

Possible Causes

Viral infections can take hold when the immune system is weakened due to stress. Toxic overload can also be a contributing factor. At an emotional level, can be caused by feelings that your life lacks joy.

Other Suggestions

Take the time to draw love to yourself and love those who are around you. Affirm that your life is full of joy.

Echinacea is anti-viral and can help the body deal with the invading microbes. The herb astragalus has good immune boosting properties. Take one teaspoon of dried astragalus steeped in a cup of just boiled water with honey three times a day.

Rest and drink plenty of fluids. Eat lightly. Eliminate processed foods from the diet. Take 2,000-4,000 mg of vitamin C daily. Add raw garlic to your diet. Traditional Chinese medicine can help viral infections.

11 Chronic Conditions

Angina

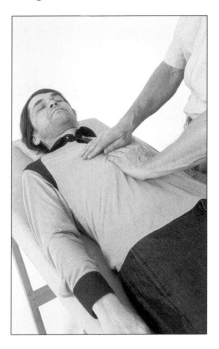

15-MINUTE TREATMENT

Treat the heart directly by placing one hand over the heart itself and one hand over the diaphragm, forming a T-shape. Treat the foot area to bring the energy down to the feet as well as the shoulder area (Position 12).

Possible Causes

Factors that contribute to heart disease include poor diet, a sedentary lifestyle, being over-weight, plus smoking. A recent study in the journal *Health Psychology* suggests that anger and high hostility levels could mean you have a greater chance of developing heart disease. Other factors include a lack of love and joy in your life.

Other Suggestions

Include plenty of organic vegetables and fruit in your diet. Ensure you are eating what is right for your system. Check out the book *Eat Right for Your Type* by Dr Peter D'Adamo, who has successfully treated a number of people with angina. Make regular exercise part of your life. Begin gently and, if the angina surfaces, stop immediately. Supplement the diet with hawthorn, coenzyme Q10, L-carnitine and magnesium.

Delay is the best remedy. Take a few deep breaths when you feel an episode rising. Quietly observe it without suppressing it. If you feel you are becoming angry, express it safely by screaming or beating a pillow to release the pent-up emotion. Meditation can do much to calm the mind. Nurture yourself and those close to you. Ask 'What can I do to bring more love into my life today?'

Arthritis

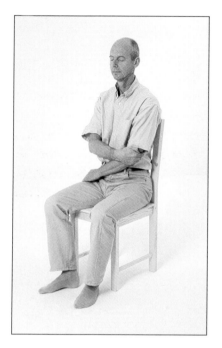

15-MINUTE TREATMENT

Treat the areas that are affected directly by placing one hand above and the other below the joint. For self-treatment, place one hand above the joint. Then change and treat below the joint. A whole-body treatment is desirable if time is available.

Possible Causes

Arthritis often arises when a person feels unloved. As a result, a person becomes inflexible and rigid in their approach, levelling criticism at others.

Other Suggestions

Draw love into your life. By nurturing and approving of yourself and others, you can choose to love and be loved. This allows more joy and spontaneity into your life.

The best anti-inflammatory supplements are omega-3 fats found in oily fish. Eating fish three times a week, supplemented with fish-oil capsules, will help reduce joint pain. Keep the joints flexible without stressing them. Swimming is ideal. Try a form of aerobic yoga called psychocalisthenics. More information on this can be found at the psychocalisthenics website listed on page 196.

Asthma

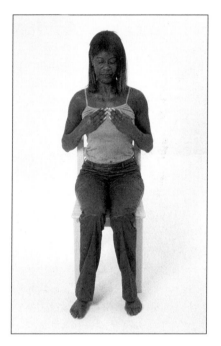

15-MINUTE TREATMENT

Place both hands directly over the lungs. Also treat the heart and solar plexus (Positions 5 and 6). Treat the upper and lower back (Positions 13 and 14).

Possible Causes

Sometimes caused by a feeling of being emotionally stifled or suppressed. A child can sometimes unwittingly be made to feel helpless by being over-mothered.

Other Suggestions

It is important to ensure that clear boundaries are put in place so that the asthma sufferer feels powerful and in control. Ayurvedic medicine can be helpful.

Blood Pressure

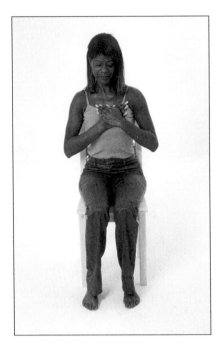

15-MINUTE TREATMENT

Treat the heart directly, one hand over the other (Position 5).

Possible Causes

Stress, a poor diet and a sedentary lifestyle are all factors that contribute to high blood pressure. At an emotional level, it may be caused by anger and frustration. This may be due to unresolved emotional problems.

Other Suggestions

Dietary changes can assist the lowering of blood pressure. Losing weight and giving up smoking can, too. However, the biggest changes may need to come from within. Psychotherapy can be helpful in getting to the root of deeply-held resentment and unresolved issues, as well as assisting with stress-management. Meditation can encourage the calming of the mind. Non-competitive sports are an ideal way to let off steam.

Bronchitis

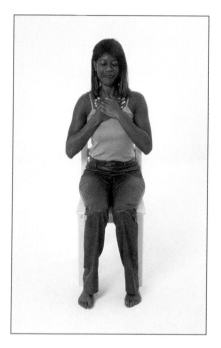

15-MINUTE TREATMENT

Place the hands at the top of the chest, below the throat. Then treat the heart, solar plexus and abdomen area (Positions 5 to 7).

Possible Causes

Smoking and pollution cause infection of the bronchi. Poor diet and lack of exercise also contribute. Can also result from working or living in an emotionally-charged environment. This condition arises when the system becomes overloaded with toxins.

Other Suggestions

A healing space needs to be created where peace and harmony prevail. Traditional Chinese Medicine has effective remedies to cleanse the body, such as the herbs mulberry bark, astragalus root, cinnamon twig and dried ginger. They are prescribed on an individual basis depending on symptoms. Meditation can help to calm the mind.

Cancer

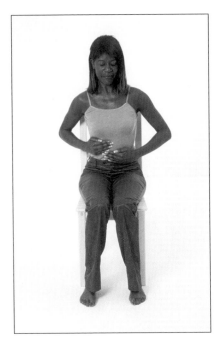

15-MINUTE TREATMENT

Treat the area of discomfort directly. Give whole-body treatments as often as possible. Place one hand on the liver and the other on the spleen, as shown in the photograph, to boost the immune system.

Possible Causes

There are many kinds of cancer, with different causes. Can be due to environmental factors or heredity. At an emotional level, cancer can be caused by long-standing resentment. Ask yourself if there is anyone you need to forgive.

Other Suggestions

Depending on the kind of cancer, the first step is to eliminate cancer-stimulating agents such as a high-fat diet, smoking, too much sun exposure, alcohol and pesticides. Then build up the immune system with diet and supplements. Cut out fried foods. Increase your intake of antioxidant foods such as organically-grown broccoli, carrots, tomatoes, watercress, cauliflower, berries, grapes, lemon, tuna and salmon. Drink plenty of water. Take vitamin supplements of A, C and E. Visit a naturopath or nutritionist, who will be able to create a personalized, healing diet for you.

Reiki can be helpful in supporting treatment. It is recommended before and after radiotherapy to strengthen and support the body's healing processes.

There isn't any one cause of cancer, and there are many cures. Deepak Chopra believes it is possible to attain a state of bliss, where healing can take place. In his book *Perfect Health*, he describes a study of over 400 people whose symptoms went into spontaneous remission. They had all found a different way to heal, whether it was through a particular diet, mega-vitamin therapy or other treatments. Diverse strategies emerged, but all reported eventually moving into a space where fear, despair and sickness were nonexistent.

If you feel you might be carrying any resentment for anything that has happened in the past, choose to release it and forgive. Fill your world with joy. Work through any issues you may have with a counsellor or therapist. Contact the Bristol Cancer Care Clinic or the Bernie Siegel's Mind–Body Wellness Centre (website details on page 195). The Internet is excellent for research. Find out how you can create your own miracle.

Cholesterol

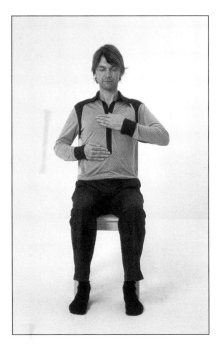

15-MINUTE TREATMENT

Treat the heart area directly with one hand, and the other on the liver. Also treat the solar plexus, the abdomen and back of the heart (Positions 5 to 7 and 13).

Possible Causes

Raised cholesterol levels can be attributed to poor diet, weight problems and a sedentary lifestyle. Heredity can also be a contributing factor. At an emotional level, this condition can be due to the inability to feel joy flowing through you. Fear may be the underlying cause.

Other Suggestions

Make changes to your lifestyle so that you nurture your body. Make sure you choose to nourish yourself with plenty of organic vegetables and fruits. Make exercise a regular part of your life. Supplement the diet with coenzyme Q10, ginkgo biloba, hawthorn, plus vitamin B complex and magnesium. Open yourself fully to enjoy life and all that it brings.

Chronic Fatigue Syndrome (ME)

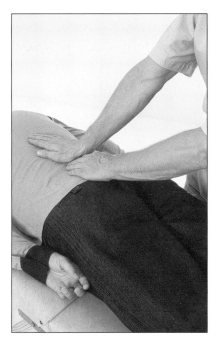

15-MINUTE TREATMENT

Treat the head positions, heart, solar plexus and pelvic region (Positions 1 to 6 and 8). Treat the lower back with both hands pointing towards the head. A full-body treatment is advised as often as possible for this condition.

Possible Causes

Over-achievers are often affected by this illness. Can be caused by sufferers' failing to meet their own needs, while making considerable efforts to please others. Fear of change could be an issue. There could be repression. Ask yourself how you would ideally choose to spend time. Be honest. Be prepared to make major changes.

Other Suggestions

Affirm your willingness to change, knowing it will be safe for you to do so. Traditional Chinese Medicine can be helpful. Chinese remedies containing herbs such as ginseng and ginkgo biloba have significant therapeutic value and many work on conditions for which Western doctors have no drugs or treatment. High doses of vitamin C (around 3,000 mg per day) are recommended, as well as including garlic in your diet. Psychotherapy would be beneficial.

Deep Vein Thrombosis (DVT)

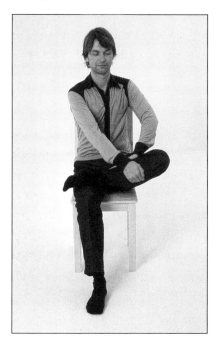

15-MINUTE TREATMENT

Treat the legs where affected, and also the heart area to boost the circulation (Position 5).

Possible Causes

DVT can be caused when a person spends a long period without being able to move around. This could result from time spent sitting at a computer or from travelling on a long-haul flight. The metaphysical cause reflects the closing-down of the flow of joy through your system. Make sure you embrace life fully.

Other Suggestions

If you must spend a long period sitting down in a confined space, be sure to do leg and foot exercises as frequently as you can. Press the balls of your feet down hard against the floor and lift your heels to help increase the blood flow in your legs and prevent clotting. Get up and walk around as much as possible. Breathing exercises can improve the circulation. Drink plenty of water. Avoid sleeping pills. Take advantage of refuelling stopovers where it is possible to leave the aircraft. Frequent flyers may try wearing compression socks (available from most pharmacies). If you experience uncomfortable leg pain during a flight, see a doctor.

See also Chapter 12, page 138.

Depression

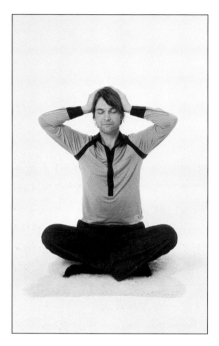

15-MINUTE TREATMENT

Treat the sides of the head as shown. Treat the eyes, the temples and the back of the head (Positions 1, 2 and 3) as well as treating the heart directly by placing one hand over the heart and the other across the chest, forming a T-shape. Also, treat the solar plexus (Position 6).

Possible Causes

There are many causes. Grief is one. It can sometimes be caused by deep-rooted anger which has been turned inwards rather than expressed.

Other Suggestions

Some experts believe that the key to depression does not lie in limiting the capacity to feel emotions. By intensifying the feelings, the healing system can be activated. In other words, developing a passion for something can be just as intensive as feelings of despair, and absorbing in a much more positive way.

Place a strict time-limit on negative thinking – for example 10 minutes in the morning and 10 minutes in the evening. Ask yourself how your day would be if you were happy. What would you do if you felt happiness flow through you? If Dr Usui were alive today, he would probably add a sixth principle: 'Just for today, choose to be happy.' If a person pretends to be happy, it soon becomes genuine. Read Robert Holden's book *Happiness Now*.

Aerobic exercise is excellent for depression. Make sure your posture is upright. Keep your head up and look straight ahead or around you. It is impossible to feel despondent when you're walking tall. It is surprising what a difference this makes.

The herbal treatment St John's Wort is a natural mood-enhancer and helps to regulate disturbed sleep cycles. Psychotherapy can help relieve symptoms. Cut out processed foods, sugar and all stimulants such as tea, coffee, chocolate and fizzy drinks. A nutritionist can help identify factors which can be corrected by dietary changes or supplementation.

Reiki can be helpful to relieve anxiety and enhance emotional well-being. It can help you to overcome this condition.

Eczema

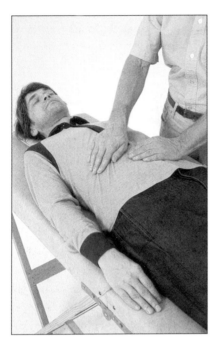

15-MINUTE TREATMENT

Place your hands across the forehead area. Treat the solar plexus and abdomen (Positions 6 and 7) as well as the shoulder blades and lower back (Positions 13 and 14). Treat away from the body where the skin is broken.

Possible Causes

Poor diet and stress contribute to this condition. At an emotional level, a sufferer may feel resentment from others. It could also indicate a need to release long-standing issues.

Other Suggestions

Traditional Chinese Medicine is helpful. Recent studies in the *Lancet* and the *British Journal of Dermatology* have shown that the Chinese herbal preparation Zemaphyte could help eczema. Digestive enzymes such as bromelain help to improve the digestion so that more nutrients are absorbed. Evening primrose oil can provide essential fatty acids. Creams made with anti-inflammatory essential oils such as yarrow and camomile can soothe the skin. To ease the effects of conventional medications, eat foods rich in vitamin C, such as fresh vegetables and fruits.

Nurture yourself in harmonious surroundings. Ensure your relationships are not draining you. Start a journal to express your feelings. Surround yourself with caring, supportive friends. Allow yourself to feel safe, secure and at peace with the world.

Epilepsy

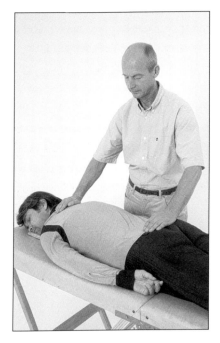

15-MINUTE TREATMENT

Treat the solar plexus and the abdomen area (Positions 6 and 7). Turn the person over and place one hand at the base of the spine and the other at the top of the spine. In our experience, the head of an epileptic is too sensitive to treat.

Possible Causes

Poor diet, stress and alcohol are all said to be causes of epilepsy, although in the majority of cases the cause is unknown. At an emotional level it can occur when there is repression or a rejection of some aspect of yourself, which you are not comfortable with. Sometimes there is a subconscious rejection of life itself, or a feeling of struggle.

Other Suggestions

Cut out the known triggers such as alcohol and stress, and make regular exercise part of your life. Gentle, non-invasive body work, such as trager or feldenkrais, can help with stress-reduction. (For further information, see Trager UK and the Feldenkrais Guild on page 196.) Choose to see life as joyful. Self-acceptance and self-love can be powerfully healing.

Glandular Fever

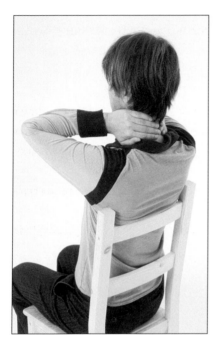

15-MINUTE TREATMENT

Place hands either side of the throat, fingers touching at the back of the neck. Treat the jaw line and throat area (Position 4). Then place one hand across the base of the throat and the other on the upper chest. Also treat the armpits, solar plexus and abdomen area (Positions 6 and 7).

Possible Causes

The body is attempting to eliminate accumulated toxins. At an emotional level, this may be a result of feelings of anger at not being appreciated enough or valued. Can also reflect a lack of self-love.

Other Suggestions

Traditional Chinese Medicine assists elimination and strengthens the immune system. Homoeopathy can help relieve symptoms. Suggested remedies are *Argentum nitricum*, *Digitalis purpurea* and *Astacus fluviatilis*. For more information contact ABC Homeopathy (contact details on page 195).

Rest and take plenty of liquids to keep the body hydrated. Affirm self-love and appreciation of your uniqueness. Ensure your life is balanced with enough time and space to meet your needs. Recognize when you are becoming stressed and pace yourself, knowing there is time for everything.

Hay Fever

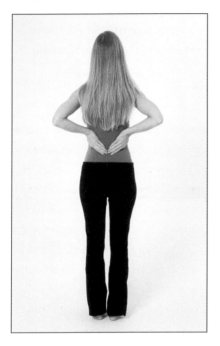

15-MINUTE TREATMENT

Treat all the head positions (Positions 1 to 4). Also treat the kidneys, as shown in the photograph.

Possible Causes

Hay fever is caused by the immune system over-reacting to environmental agents which, in themselves, are not intrinsically harmful. The immune system becomes weakened. At another level it can occur when a person becomes emotionally congested and energetically depleted.

Other Suggestions

Take measures to strengthen your immune system well before the hay fever season begins. Cut out foods that cause dampness, phlegm and spleen damage. Eliminate wheat, dairy and sugary products. Have a personalized tincture made up for you by a Chinese herbal practitioner. This will desensitize the system and reduce symptoms. Exercise for 20 minutes a day, getting the heart going. Relax deeply for a short period each day (sitting in front of the television is not enough). There are some excellent relaxation CDs available. The website www.newworldmusic.com offers a good choice. A course in acupuncture will be of great benefit. Deepak Chopra also recommends a self-massage with sesame oil before showering each day, to stimulate the immune system.

At an emotional level, let go of any fear and anger that you are carrying. If you feel yourself becoming too agitated, visualize a positive outcome.

HIV (AIDS)

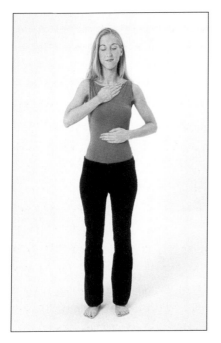

15-MINUTE TREATMENT

Place one hand on the thymus gland (chest area) and the other on the spleen to boost the immune system. Treat the pelvic area (Position 8) to release feelings of insecurity. Treat the back of the head (Position 3) to relieve anxiety and depression. A full-body treatment will further strengthen the system and improve physical, mental and spiritual well-being. If you have the virus, Reiki training is recommended so you can give yourself a treatment as often as possible.

Possible Causes

There is considerable diversity of scientific opinion about where HIV comes from. Emotionally it may result from feeling powerless and defenceless. Believing nobody cares. Thinking you are not good enough. Sexual guilt. Feeling unimportant and worthless.

Other Suggestions

Have a personalized tincture made up by a practitioner of Traditional Chinese Medicine to relieve symptoms and boost the immune system.

A group of people who are HIV-positive have taken Reiki training in conjunction with other natural healing methods as a means of prompting their bodies to respond to the virus and cope with the stress of the virus. At the time of writing it is not known how helpful Reiki has been. What is known is that there are more long-term survivors of the virus than ever before. The majority of these people have incorporated holistic nutrition and natural healing methods into their lives. Whether the long-term survivors were affected with a less virulent strain of HIV, which they developed immunity to, or their immune systems have been strengthened by their holistic endeavours is not yet known.

Accept yourself for the incredible person that you are. Allow yourself to feel loved, powerful and capable. Affirm that you are part of the incredible universal design.

Irritable Bowel Syndrome (IBS)

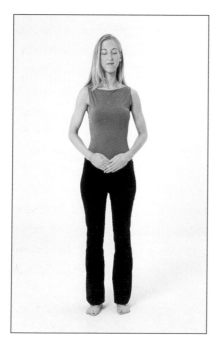

15-MINUTE TREATMENT

Place your hands directly over the area of discomfort. If more time is available, treat the whole abdomen area intensively, by placing one hand on top of the other as shown in the photograph.

Possible Causes

The term IBS is used to describe a number of symptoms including diarrhoea, constipation, abdominal pain and indigestion. There are many contributory causes to this condition including food allergy, stress, toxic overload, infection and overactive gut muscles.

This condition can cause the intestines to work overtime. The job of the intestines is to break down everything into small packages, rather like a general sorting office. At an emotional level, ask yourself if you are over-analysing situations in your life. This might be reflected in the body. If your mind is working overtime, so might your intestines. Choose to trust in your 'gut feeling' and have positive expectations of the outcome.

Other Suggestions

Eat what you know you can digest. Your system may have become overloaded and sensitive. A nutritionist can determine whether symptoms can be relieved by dietary changes or whether you need supplements to help detoxify the body. Consider a nutritionist who uses a bioresonance technique to detect intolerances. Peter D'Adamo's book *Eat Right for Your Type* may be helpful in determining the right foods for you.

Hypnotherapy can be helpful. Visit a hypnotherapist or obtain an audio course designed to alleviate IBS (see Hypnotherapy Home Audio Courses on page 196).

Alternatively, you can combine Reiki with hypnotherapy and make your own unique recording that will stimulate your body's own healing mechanism. An example can be found on page 190.

Migraine

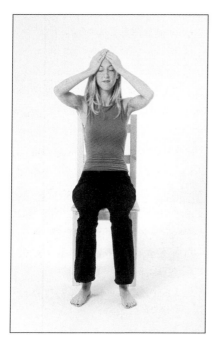

15-MINUTE TREATMENT

At the first sign of a migraine, treat the eyes, temples and back of head (Positions 1, 2 and 3) as well as across the top of the head. Also treat the solar plexus area (Position 6). When treating others, treat directly over the area of discomfort.

Possible Causes

Stress is a major factor. Deep-rooted anger or other strong emotions can contribute, as can feeling overwhelmed by information or too much pressure on your time.

Other Suggestions

When it comes to migraine, we are speaking from direct experience. Chris used to suffer from migraines before taking Reiki. The following are suggestions which stopped his attacks.

Identify the stressors in your life and deal with them. Take stress-management seriously (if necessary, obtain help from a therapist or life-coach). Acupuncture is helpful for relieving energetic blockages. Check your diet, removing any foods that may cause an attack. Keep off known trigger foods such as cheese, red wine, chocolate, MSG (monosodium glutamate, commonly found in processed foods) and peanuts. Ensure you drink plenty of water and never let yourself become dehydrated. Take vigorous outdoor exercise that is non-competitive, and make time for relaxation.

Repetitive Strain Injury (RSI)

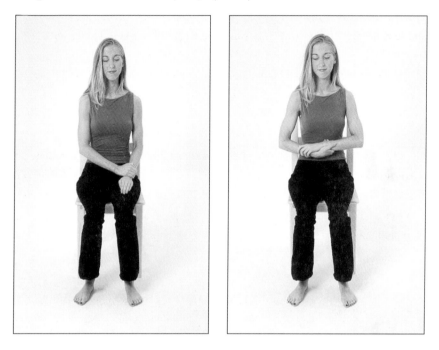

15-MINUTE TREATMENT

Place your hand around your wrist or the area most affected, as shown. When treating others, place both hands around the injury. Also, treat the elbows and the hands. If more time is available, treat the eyes, temples and back of the head (Positions 1 to 3).

Possible Causes

The most common form of RSI is carpal tunnel syndrome, which affects the wrists, hands and sometimes the lower arms. This is usually brought on by overuse of the wrists in an incorrect position. This syndrome is often suffered by computer-users and keyboard-players. At an emotional level, RSI represents lack of movement and ease. It can indicate anger and frustration at injustice.

Other Suggestions

Hot and cold applications can help, as can gentle massage with arnica cream. Sufferers are often deficient in vitamin B6 and calcium. Take supplements of 50 mg B6 and 400 mg calcium at each meal. A combination of acupuncture, osteopathy and Reiki can alleviate this condition. Opt for new thought-patterns affirming that you handle all your experiences with wisdom, love and ease.

Rheumatism

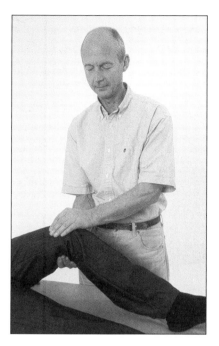

15-MINUTE TREATMENT

Sandwich the affected joint with both hands. Treat the temples and the back of the head (Positions 2 and 3). Then move down to the solar plexus, abdomen and pelvic region (Positions 6 to 8).

Possible Causes

This condition can affect the most positive of people, but is sometimes caused by feeling unloved and even victimized. There could be a tendency to harbour resentment, causing a build-up of toxic emotions.

Other Suggestions

The herbal remedy feverfew can help to alleviate the symptoms. Dietary changes can moderate the inflammation. Bee-sting therapy has also been known to be helpful. Drink kombucha several times a day and fast on vegetable juices and warm vegetable broth regularly to detoxify the system. Consult a naturopath for specific advice.

Love and approve of yourself and others. Acknowledge you create your own experience. Feel free to enjoy every moment of your life.

Sciatica

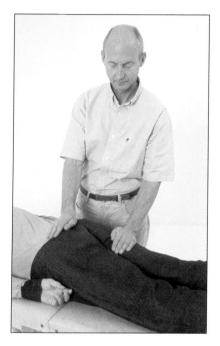

15-MINUTE TREATMENT

Treat the lower back, the base of the spine and the soles of the feet (Positions 14, 15 and 16). Place one hand on the base of the spine and the other on the top of one thigh at the point where the legs join the body. Change to treat the other thigh. Treat the back of the knees.

Possible Causes

Stress is a contributing factor. Other factors can include financial concerns and fear of an uncertain future. There may be a sense of feeling unduly pressurized by a situation, a relationship or too many commitments.

Other Suggestions

Relax completely. Trust that your future needs will be met. Acknowledge that you create firm foundations for yourself and your life. Affirm that all your experiences are handled with wisdom, love and with ease.

John Sarno, a New York doctor, believes that most back pain is the result of the mind's interference with the normal functioning of nerves and blood circulation to muscles. Understanding how the mind produces pain has brought relief to many of his patients (see Books for Superhealth on page 193).

Unresolved emotional issues and stressful situations can cause pain to manifest. Ask yourself if there are any issues that you need to deal with. Good stress-management plus acupuncture, visualization, healthy foods and supplements can transform the situation.

12 First Aid and Prevention

FIRST AID

Broken Bones

It is essential that the injured person sees a doctor as soon as possible. In an emergency, the person can be helped with Reiki while awaiting assistance. Place one hand on the forehead and the other at the back of the head. This will have a calming effect. Do not give any Reiki to the area of the fracture until a doctor has treated it. After this, Reiki can help to accelerate healing by treating the site of the fracture several times a day.

Burns

This advice is for minor household burns. For anything more serious, the injured person must be taken immediately to a doctor for emergency treatment.

Cool immediately with cold running water. If the skin is unbroken and you have an aloe vera plant, apply the sap from the leaves directly on to the area. Where the skin has broken, cover with a sterile, non-stick material. Give Reiki above and to the sides of the burn, keeping the hands a little higher than usual.

Insect Bites

To help reduce itching and inflammation, apply 1 drop of peppermint oil directly onto the bite. Peppermint has antiseptic and anti-inflammatory properties. Alternatively, echinacea tincture is helpful, applied similarly. The homoeopathic remedy apis mellifica is recommended for bee stings or insect bites. Immediately treat with Reiki, keeping your hands above the injured area.

Sprains

Apply ice to the affected area. Treat with Reiki as soon as possible. Take the homoeopathic remedy byronia to reduce swelling. Arnica tincture is also helpful for shock. Tubular bandages can be helpful for support.

Whiplash Injuries

Apply an ice-pack to the injured area for up to 20 minutes at a time every hour. After 24 hours use ice-packs or heat to relieve the discomfort. Hot showers may help. It may be more comfortable sleeping on a roll-shaped pillow positioned behind the neck. Treat with Reiki as often as possible. Take anti-inflammatory devil's claw or green-lipped mussel, plus a multi-vitamin with minerals and calcium. A chiropractor or osteopath may help.

Wounds

Bandage or wrap the wound in the usual way. For all types of small wounds, give Reiki immediately for about 15 minutes. Keep your hands directly above without making skin contact. In cases of strong bleeding, go immediately for emergency treatment.

PREVENTION

Deep Vein Thrombosis

DVT has been in the news due to the controversy surrounding long-haul flights. However, it is possible to suffer a blood clot in the legs from sitting too long at a computer. For further information, see DVT in Chapter 11 (page 113).

- Request the seats alongside the emergency exit doors, as they have more legroom. (It is not a good idea to say you have an injury, as people without mobility difficulties must take these seats).
- Travel in business class if you can afford to do so. At the time of writing, many airlines are offering the equivalent at bargain prices, so it may be worth enquiring.
- Avoid boarding a long-haul flight while sleep-deprived or exhausted.
- Keep as active as you can during the flight, getting up and moving around as often as possible.
- Avoid in-flight meals that are rich in saturated fats: Avoid butter pats, slabs of cheddar cheese, rich creamy sauces or fried breakfast dishes. Have lighter options, if available, such as salmon or chicken in a low-fat sauce. Snack on raw fruit and vegetables that are water-rich. Unless the airline objects, bring your own.
- Avoid sleeping tablets, as taking them would leave you confined with little movement for a long period.
- Give Reiki to your heart.
- Exercise the leg and foot muscles as often as you can.
- During any stopovers, leave the aircraft and walk around.
- Drink plenty of water and keep active.

Jet Lag

To minimize the effects there are a few measures you can take before you fly:

- Adapt the body's sleeping pattern to the time zone you will be travelling to, several days before you depart.
- As an anti-stress measure, take a time-release 1,000-mg vitamin C and a high-potency B vitamin before the flight.
- Try to book a flight that lands at 9 p.m. at your destination so you can get a good night's sleep after you arrive.
- Give yourself Reiki while travelling. Treat the stomach area to aid digestion, and the head positions to help you sleep. Giving yourself Reiki after you land will help you to adjust to the new time zone.

Sars Virus and Similar Bugs

The risk of contracting SARS (Severe Acute Respiratory Syndrome) is extremely low. However, it is helpful to be aware of how you can protect yourself. Here are some suggestions:

- Avoid non-essential travel to areas badly hit by the virus.
- Build up good body immunity. Give yourself Reiki on a regular basis for at least two weeks before departing. Take the immune-system-boosting astragalus, plus a good multivitamin, for a couple of weeks before your trip. Continue while travelling and for a further 10 days after your return.
- Be sure you are not exhausted at the time of travel.
- Keep yourself physically active, eat well and have plenty of rest.
- Wash your hands frequently and maintain good personal hygiene.
- Avoid contact with large numbers of people or places with poor ventilation.
- Consider wearing a surgical mask when you are around someone who may have SARS or similar.
- Wash hands with alcohol wipes after touching infected people or objects touched by them.

Preventing Viral Infections

Some guidelines to prevent infection by a virus:

- Avoid touching your eyes or nose, where viruses take hold.
- Wash your hands regularly, especially if you have been travelling on public transport. Use disposable towels for drying hands.
- Always wash your hands before giving yourself a Reiki treatment.
- Try to avoid the company of anyone who has a bad cold.
- If someone with a bad cold or virus does come round to your home, spray surfaces afterwards with a disinfectant to prevent it spreading.
- Make sure family members with respiratory tract infections use paper handkerchiefs, and dispose of them carefully.
- Keep healthy. Make sure you get enough sleep. Use relaxation techniques to beat stress and give yourself regular Reiki treatments.

For more information on treating viral infections, see Chapter 10 (page 68).

Using Reiki to
Transform Your Life

PART THREE

13 Reiki for a Brand New You

It is never too late to be what you might have been.
GEORGE ELIOT

As well as healing physical symptoms, Reiki can help you bring more balance and harmony into your life. Fragmented modern-day living often leaves many people feeling energetically depleted and disempowered. We juggle many roles daily. Much of our time is spent meeting other people's needs and, all too often, we lose sight of our own. I would now like you to focus your attention on a very special person. That person is you.

As you are reading this book, the chances are that you are the kind of person who wants to enhance your life. We are about to embark on a journey to help you make your life even better than it is now. Reiki can assist in this process. Our thoughts are extremely powerful and our outer reality conforms to our beliefs. This is why it is so important to think positively at all times. Energy follows thought. You are manifesting right now with your thoughts and feelings, just as you always have done. The frequency you send out acts like a magnet, attracting what you put out for. Ensure you choose your thoughts carefully and consider your choices wisely.

Reiki brings you into alignment with the highest, wisest part of you, so you can manifest all that your heart desires. By allowing yourself to trust your inner guidance system, you can move closer to your dreams. To manifest, ensure you include whatever it is you want into your thoughts and beliefs. If, for example, you want to bring more love into your life, become the most loving person around. Don't focus on the lack of love. If you want to attract more abundance, become the most generous person around, so that you change your frequency to one of prosperity. Even if you are giving away the simplest cake or the smallest pot of homemade jam, allow yourself to feel generous and abundant, so your vibration alters.

Deciding to change your life begins with making a personal choice. All too often we become caught up in the reasons why we cannot do things differently, and forget just who is in charge. To enable you to create the life that you want, in the next four chapters we will show you four strategies to strengthen and support you. As you progress through them, you will learn to:

1. Restore your energy
2. Harness your inner power
3. Surround yourself with supportive, high-energy people
4. Nurture your spiritual well-being

14 Restore Your Energy

Every action you take involves using your energy. Sometimes energy is depleted when you don't take action. Your intent to do or say something can weigh heavily on your mind, and energetically drain you. Furthermore, your energy can be tethered to a situation long after the event.

Relationships can drain your energy, as can living in an environment not conducive to your state of mind. Not eating a high enough quality of fresh, natural foods can, too. Depletion can result from working in an environment that doesn't allow you to express your creativity, or from having financial concerns that haven't been addressed.

IDENTIFY WHERE THE ENERGY GOES

The first step is to identify where energy is being drained. Then it is possible to re-organize yourself so that you are building and not diminishing your energy reserves.

Here are a few questions to start you off:

- Are there relationships in my life that are draining me?
- Are there phone calls I should make, letters or e-mails I should send?
- Is there an unresolved conflict with anyone – either in the workplace, within my family or among my friends?
- Is there a relationship I should bring to an end?
- Is there a gap for someone special in my life?
- Is there a shortage of high-energy people to spend time with?
- Is there a project I need to bring to completion?

- Is there anyone I need to forgive?
- Is my car due for maintenance or repair?
- Is my home cluttered and disorganized?
- Are there repairs I need to make?
- Are there financial concerns I need to give my attention to?

Make a list of the areas in which your energy is being drained. Make it as comprehensive as possible.

REPLENISH THE ENERGY BANKS

Now, create an action plan to deal with the items and decide how the list can be tackled. Some suggestions are:

- Decide to take personal action immediately and cross it off the list.
- Delegate it to someone else, who can take care of it without your input.
- Bring in hired help or get a family member to sort it out.
- Decide not to take further action by disposing of the item needing attention.
- Give away, recycle or replace anything that requires excessive maintenance.
- Ask others for help with difficult tasks that require a particular expertise.
- Put a time-limit on your plan, so that everything is dealt with quickly.

If you've done the Second Degree Reiki course, you can use the absent-healing procedure to energize the action plan. Otherwise, set the intent that you would like all the items on your list dealt with quickly and easily. Hold the list in your hands and visualize a flow of energy from your hands empowering the list, speeding up the process.

CLEAR CLUTTER

Melanie works at the airport in a stressful management role that often leaves her feeling depleted. She found she had little time for herself and limited energy left for relaxing with her two children during weekends and evenings.

Melanie realized that one of the major energy-drains in her life was the clutter that had piled up in her home. Clearing it would require a great deal of effort and, on top of this, she doesn't like to waste useful items. Melanie admitted that she didn't like to throw things away and had a tendency to hoard things.

On top of her own possessions and the children's clutter there was her ex-husband's paraphernalia and the belongings of a late, beloved aunt. At one point Melanie could not walk around her bedroom because these things covered the entire floor space. The situation began to get her down. Melanie decided she must be ruthless in disposing of everything she and her children could not use. She gave away many items to friends and to charity. When no more could be recycled, she took the difficult decision to throw the rest away.

Melanie felt fantastic once her house was tidy and uncluttered. She felt energized and calm. It is amazing how liberated you feel when your energy banks are replenished. Melanie decided she would keep her home clutter-free and surround herself with uplifting items.

Clearing clutter is a powerful way to leave the past behind. We all accumulate many belongings over the years. Disposing of them can become a major problem. There are some excellent books on simplifying your life, and nearly all advise clearing out everything you are not using right now.

When you have cleared your home, you will feel wonderful. Be ruthless and get rid of anything you have not used, repaired or worn for the last couple of years or more. If you are uncertain about something, box it. Date the box 12 months from now. If you still haven't used the contents by then, get rid of it.

ENERGIZE YOUR HOME

After clearing the rooms in your home, clear the stale energy with Reiki. Open the windows wide, sweep the floors, clean the surfaces, turn off any electrical appliances and give the room an energetic boost by visualizing light coming out of your hands and filling the room with life-force energy. For those who have Second Degree Reiki training, send energy to the room using the technique taught at that level. If you haven't, you can still set the intent for the room to be cleansed and energized. Bring some fresh flowers in, perhaps light a scented candle or play some music, and relax.

If you feel the energy in the room needs even more of a boost, you may decide to redecorate. Choose colours that soothe and uplift you. Use eco-friendly paints, free of toxic chemicals which can cause irritation and allergies (see page 198 for suppliers).

Moving to a new home may mean that you wish to clear the atmosphere left by previous occupants. Feng shui experts suggest placing a dish of salt in each room for several hours to absorb any negative energy. Remove and dispose of the salt. Then bring some fresh flowers into your home. Following this, energetically cleanse the room with Reiki as before. You may also want to energize some bottled spring water with a few drops of your favourite essential oil (lemon is refreshing). Place your hands on the bottle to infuse with Reiki energy for a few moments, then scatter some of the water in each room. Having cleansed the rooms, choose to place only uplifting items in them, and enjoy your living space.

If you find it difficult to begin, give yourself a Reiki treatment with the intent that your home is effortlessly cleared. Treat the head positions. This will help to energize the process.

When clutter has been cleared physically from your home and mentally from your mind, you are able to restore your life-energy. The space created allows you to focus on areas that you have long wanted to give your attention but haven't been able to.

BRING BACK ENERGY FROM OLD SITUATIONS AND EVENTS

Carole is a singer and songwriter. Her music reflects many of the interesting periods in her life, when she lived in various parts of the United States. She now lives in England where she enjoys a very different life with her new partner in a suburb of Manchester.

Carole told me that, while she mostly felt happy and content, her energy seemed to be all over the place. She felt as if it were tied up in all different places, experiences and challenges in her life. Carole decided to 'recall' the energy. She began to take a journey back in time to all the significant moments in her life. Whenever she homed in on an event that had affected her emotionally, she called the energy back by saying 'I call back the energy from ... (whatever the situation was).' Eventually she brought the energy back from every instance in which she felt she had been emotionally affected. It was a powerful exercise and she said she felt terrific afterwards. Allowing herself to revisit situations enabled her to release attachment. Afterwards she felt freer and more alive than she had for a long time.

Can you think of a time in your life that had such an impact that you are still affected by it today? You may have some energy to recall. Such instances could be recent or may have happened many years ago. They could be major events or a hurtful comment that has taken on a life of its own.

If you feel you have energy to recall, give yourself a Reiki treatment focusing on the head and heart area. During your session take a journey back in time and make a note of significant events that occurred. After your treatment, continue to focus on times when you responded with strong emotions, as well as those times when you wish you had. Sometimes we put our anger or grief on hold and there is still energy tied up in the situation. Make a note of each one. Then call the energy back. Continue until you have dealt with each significant event. Congratulate yourself for the action you have taken, and then relax.

Significant events in my life are:

....

....

....

....

....

....

....

....

....

....

'I call back energy from...'

15 Harness Your Inner Power

Much of the work in the last chapter has concentrated on consolidating your energy. This is important, as it gives you a powerful base from which to move forward. It is helpful at this stage to look at the people in your life and consider whether there is anyone you need to forgive. Anger and blame hold us back and keep us disempowered. While Buddhists believe that suffering is an inevitable part of the human condition, forgiveness is the key to liberation. A Native American expression says if there is an enemy in your heart, it is not safe there for a friend.

FORGIVE AND FORGET

If there is someone you need to forgive, remember the following:

- It is important to recognize that your pain is coming from the hurt feelings, thoughts and physical upset you are suffering *now*, not then.
- It can help to share your pain with others and benefit from their support.
- Do whatever you need to do to feel better. Forgiveness is for you alone.
- Forgiving is neither about forgetting nor condoning what happened.
- Forgiveness does not necessarily mean reconciliation with the person who upset you. It is about finding peace within yourself.
- Remember, you do not need the other person to admit they were wrong or that they wronged you before you make the decision to forgive.
- Choosing to have compassion for yourself and whoever wronged you is a powerful step.

- Forgiveness liberates you – and living a happy, fulfilled life is the best retribution.
- Treating your heart with Reiki can help to heal the pain and allow you to move forward.

LET GO

Equally, you may feel remorse for errors you have made in the past. David became consumed by guilt, because he had nearly called in to see his beloved father one Sunday morning, but decided against it at the last minute. Later that day he found out his father had suffered a fatal heart attack. David was a doctor and he knew that, had he been there, the outcome could have been different. What upset him so much was that he always visited his father on Sunday mornings and just on this occasion, he hadn't.

It is too easy to carry burdens around in our hearts. Blaming or punishing ourselves won't change the situation. Have compassion for yourself and lighten your load. Treat your heart area with Reiki.

DEVELOP UNSHAKEABLE SELF-CONFIDENCE

Many of us have been culturally conditioned to believe that thinking a lot of ourselves is wrong. As a result, we grow up undermining our achievements and never feeling completely comfortable with ourselves. This varies with different cultures, but it is certainly true in the UK, where we are quick to shrug off compliments and pass the credit for our achievements elsewhere.

In failing to give ourselves the approval we deserve, we wait for it to come from others. When this doesn't happen, we downgrade our efforts and our self-worth plummets.

Caroline is one of the kindest people you could meet. She offers to help whomever she can and will go to great lengths to give others the opportunity to improve their lives. Whenever we call round she is always worrying that her efforts are not enough. She has a happy, loving marriage and is well liked by her large family and many friends. Her kitchen is filled with party invitations and her home regularly welcomes many visitors. Yet, despite her endeavours, Caroline's self-esteem is surprisingly low. She never feels quite good enough, smart enough or kind enough. When she has a need, she keeps it to herself, because she doesn't consider her needs important enough to be met. She wouldn't want to let anyone know how exhausted she is and how much help she could do with. Underneath it all, I suspect Caroline yearns for the appreciation she deserves. Sadly, she is unlikely to receive it until she places a high enough value upon herself and her efforts.

Showing appreciation for someone can make their day, but it doesn't give them confidence if they don't possess it already. Confidence comes from within. It begins with approving of who you are, and liking yourself. Groucho Marx made the ultimate not-good-enough declaration when he joked that he was writing to his club offering his resignation, saying 'I would never join a club that would have me as a member.'

However, confidence is not about believing in yourself when everyone else does. It is the opposite. It is confidence to have self-belief when nobody else does. Below is a plan to help you to develop and maintain your confidence.

Action Plan: Blueprint for Confidence

1. You Are Unique
Take a moment to consider what makes you special.
Now write a list of your unique qualities:

....

....

....

....

....

....

Describe the character traits you would never change:

....

....

....

Give yourself Reiki with the intent that your self-confidence increases each day as you appreciate just how special you are.

2. Don't Compare Yourself to Anyone Else

Angela was unhappy because she had bought a sweater. It was the most expensive sweater she had ever purchased, but she felt she must have it because everyone would know how special it was. She knew she'd feel privileged and confident wearing it. She put it on and decided to visit her friend, who lived on a grand, country estate. When she arrived, her friend apologized for being dressed in tatty old clothes to muck out the stables. To Angela's horror, she found her friend was wearing the same sweater. What was the utmost in luxury for one person was just an old sweater to another.

Angela looked at the situation differently when we talked. She realized she had been depending on props to feel good about herself. Angela realized that if she were truly confident, she could have worn a chain-store sweater as if it were a designer garment from Paris. By comparing herself to wealthier friends, she felt poverty-stricken. In fact, she was more affluent than most, but it took this situation to make her appreciate the wealth she possessed – inside herself.

A successful businessman had low self-esteem. He refused to acknowledge his astonishing achievements because 'he knew he was a failure' compared to his clever, accomplished uncle.

Successful entrepreneurs can be daunted by unfavourable comparisons to Donald Trump or Richard Branson. Always give yourself credit for your accomplishments. Be generous. Acknowledge that YOUR efforts make a difference.

In the heart-warming film *It's A Wonderful Life*, an angel shows the main character what the world would have been like if he had never been born. James Stewart's character, George Bailey, comes to realize the power of the individual and the difference one person can make. He'd almost thrown his life away because he'd allowed a relatively minor setback to undermine his efforts. After the experience with the angel, he reassessed his priorities.

Strive to be the best that you can, but don't let your unique achievements be undermined by comparing yourself unfavourably to anyone else. Treat your solar plexus area with Reiki.

3. Always Think Positively

Refuse to allow any negative thoughts to take hold. Adopt an optimistic viewpoint. Disqualify any negative statements by adding a positive one onto it. For example, if someone says that a talk you've given could have been longer or more detailed, remind yourself that a lengthy speech could have lost the audience, and that you conveyed all the relevant points. Place your hands over your eyes and treat the area with Reiki.

4. Spend Time with Uplifting, Supportive People

The media bombards us with influences of all kinds, positive and negative. Make sure you surround yourself with uplifting, can-do influences. Listen to self-help tapes, attend inspirational lectures, read books by exceptional people who have made a difference. Spend time with loving, supportive friends who make you feel the special person that you are. Treat the back of your head with Reiki.

5. Appear Confident

Giving yourself Reiki before an event can be a terrific confidence-booster. Even when you aren't feeling particularly confident, act as if you are. By acting the part, you become it.

6. Reward Yourself

Look for ways to reward yourself when you do something that daunted you. By reinforcing the positive, your subconscious mind will help you achieve an ever better outcome next time. Let Reiki support your efforts by sending energy in advance to a successful outcome.

7. Learn from Your Mistakes

When the inevitable happens, see it as a learning experience. Self-confidence is about never letting yourself be undermined. Choose from today to have indestructible self-belief. When you learn to love and believe in yourself, you never need external approval again. You are tapping into and being sustained by your own energy source, your inner power. You will achieve self-confidence and self-reliance by generating and harvesting it.

Use Reiki to reinforce your confidence by sending energy to a successful solution next time, and trust that your inner guidance system will help you succeed.

8. Make a Difference to the World

In the film *Pay It Forward*, 11-year-old Trevor, played by Haley Joel Osment, was asked at school to think of an idea to change the world, and put it into action. He imaginatively decides to do something 'really big for three people ... something they can't do for themselves'. As the film progresses, each of these three people then do the same for three others, who continue helping three more, until countless lives are touched and changed. The film beautifully illustrates the difference one person can make.

If you think of something you can do for someone, don't hesitate. Put it into action. By choosing to help and unconditionally express love for others, everyone is enriched. If it is appropriate, offer someone a Reiki treatment. When people are touched by love, miracles happen.

9. Take Action

Make the most of every moment. Decide what is important for you, right now, and then set it in motion. See your life as a giant canvas on which you can paint your dreams.

What do you want? We have more choices today than ever before. The media attempts to tell us what we want through clever images supposedly portraying happiness. However, happiness isn't airbrushed images smiling at us from the glossy pages of *Hello!* magazine. Nor is it driving fast cars on mountain roads, as many advertisers would have us believe!

Happiness is doing what you enjoy. It is going down the path your heart wants to follow. Sometimes the yearning isn't obvious. You may have an inkling of something you have always wanted to do, but never felt you could, for one reason or another. Listen carefully for the messages from your soul. You might receive an insight during a Reiki treatment, an idea while dreaming, or inspiration walking in the park. It often whispers to you at unexpected moments.

A friend told us of a young man who came to her for coaching. As he came in, she noticed he was casually dressed, but wearing the dog collar of the clergy. When he sat down she realized she had been completely mistaken – he was wearing an ordinary shirt with a sweater on top. As he introduced himself, he explained that he had been thinking of changing his job. He was employed as a postal worker, but wanted to train as a minister. It was one of those defining moments when she knew she had been given a glimpse of the life this young man was meant to lead. He lacked confidence because of his family background. He didn't have a supportive peer group. With encouragement, he followed his heart and later trained as a priest.

As you give yourself a Reiki treatment, imagine your mind is like the sea. As well as the natural rhythm of the tides, be aware of the undercurrents. They can be likened to the subtle messages from your soul, which are accessed via your sixth sense: your intuition. Intuition is different from either impulsive or fear-based thoughts, which are loud and brash. It doesn't involve Hollywood-style images of your house burning down or that shiny, red Ferrari you've seen gleaming in the showroom window. Intuition is subtle. You may get a sense of something which just feels right (or perhaps wrong). A glimpse of a path you could take or a choice you could make. It quietly tells you something you need to know. It could be a reminder that all is not right and that it's time to do something about it. Listen carefully for those subtle messages from your soul. They are your calls to action.

Action Plan: Make Your Dreams Come True

1. Look into your heart and see if there are any unfulfilled dreams. It is never too late to try something different. Draw up a wish-list of 10 things you would like to do, try or have, if there were no limitations or restrictions of any kind. The list can contain anything at all: buying a holiday home in Tuscany, starting your own business, or taking up salsa dancing.

   ....

   ....

   ....

   ....

   ....

   ....

   ....

   ....

   ....

   ....

2. Of the 10 items, write down the three most important ones for you:

   ....

   ....

   ....

3. Once you decide what you want, take a giant leap and go for it! Next time you give yourself a Reiki treatment, set your intent for the energy to help you make your dreams come true. Believe you can accomplish anything you set your mind to, and you will.

16 Surround Yourself with Supportive, High-energy People

Stop for a moment and consider the most special, memorable times in your life. Close this book for a minute while you recall:

- What happened?
- Where were you?
- Whom were you with?

Usually such occasions will have involved spending time with people who enriched your life, making you feel confident and happy. Modern-day living is often fragmented, leaving us unable to sustain in-depth relationships. We often connect on a superficial basis while, at a deeper level, we yearn to be nurtured by more rewarding connections with others.

ARE YOUR RELATIONSHIPS UPLIFTING?

Take a closer look at your relationships. Do you feel energized and uplifted by them? Do you support each other's hopes and dreams, even though they may differ? Are you able to share your deepest feelings, including your fears as well as your passions? If a relationship leaves you feeling drained, angry, despondent or agitated, consider whether it is worth continuing.

TRACK DOWN KINDRED SPIRITS

Begin to identify people you would like to spend time with. Consider every-one you meet in your everyday life, as well as old friends. Ask yourself if they share your values and interests. What is your gut feeling about a per-son? Are they judgemental or supportive? Are they upbeat and positive, or weighed down by problems and issues? Do you feel you could connect with them at a deep level?

If you've recently taken up a new interest, you may want to join a sup-port group. Is there a course you would like to take, where you could meet like-minded others? Is there a club for hiking, skiing or sailing you could join? Whatever your interest, there will always be others who share it. Do you resonate with the people in your neighbourhood? If not, consider mov-ing nearer to people whose company you are more likely to enjoy. It could make all the difference.

ENERGIZING RELATIONSHIPS WITH REIKI

Reiki is helpful for attracting new people into your life. Before giving your-self a treatment, set the intent that you would like to meet like-minded peo-ple. Visualize yourself socializing with them.

If a relationship isn't working as well as it might, visualize Reiki ener-gy being sent for the highest good of both parties (if you have taken Reiki Second Degree training, use the absent-healing procedure). This may resolve issues energetically, but if something is not meant to last, it may hasten the end.

Ask yourself if you would like more relationships that are meaningful. Would you like to meet new friends sharing a common interest?

Do you yearn to connect with a soul mate? Make a list of the character traits you would like your new friend to have. Focusing on the list will make you aware of what qualities are important to you. Make it as detailed as possible, and then send Reiki to the list to energize it.

THE VALUE OF GOOD FRIENDS

Take time to appreciate the friends that you have. This can often strengthen the connection and move the relationship to a deeper level. We don't express enough appreciation for each other, and it can make a big difference. Rather than flattering a person, it is about acknowledging his or her special traits. Commenting on a special gift, talent or quality honours others in the highest possible way. It gives them permission to be more of who they already are.

17 Nurture Your Spiritual Well-being

Many of us struggle to find a way of living authentically in a chaotic world. The desire to express our spiritual nature is drowned by the roar of everyday life. We lose sight of our spiritual quest and disconnected from our inner wisdom.

Spiritual well-being has a different meaning for everyone. The most common elements seem to be a relationship with God, a deep sense of love, and a quest for inner peace. The most fundamental way of honouring your spiritual well-being is to live a life guided by the vision of your inner wisdom. If you can listen and act on this guidance, you will find yourself on a path that always serves your highest good.

Most people can recall a time when they wish they had made a different decision. Those times when you groan, 'I had a gut feeling I shouldn't have done that!' Intuition can often alert us to an outcome that the logical mind cannot. Many clients have told us of occasions when they had a strong feeling not to take a job or an opportunity. Reiki encourages the development of this intuitive connection with your soul or wise self.

Action Plan: Six Steps to Nurture Your Spiritual Well-being

1. Start an Inner Dialogue

Simply ask for guidance. Phrase the question in your mind and wait for a response. It may take minutes, hours or days, but the answer will present itself. It may come in the form of a dream, daydream or just as a thought. If you need to make an important decision, such as whether to end a relationship or take a new job, ask if it will serve your highest good. If you get into the habit of asking for guidance, it will soon become second nature.

Ask a question right at the beginning of a Reiki treatment. Relax and expect to receive an answer either during the session or later on.

2. Keep a Journal

This can be a helpful way of exploring feelings and spiritual desires. As well as recording your thoughts, you may want to use a journal to remember inspirational quotations, synchronistic events, spiritual experiences and other insights. A journal can be invaluable for noting dreams that would otherwise be forgotten.

Find a regular time to write in your journal, so that it becomes a special, sacred part of your day. You may want to keep the answers to self-development exercises. Keep a note of any questions you may ask, and record any replies you receive or decisions you make.

Drawing pictures can be a powerful way of accessing the subconscious mind. If you prefer not to draw, you can cut out images from magazines that appeal to you and stick them in your journal, making a large collage. Later, when you look at the compilation, you may be intrigued by what the images convey. It's surprising how expressive art allows us to be. It lets the subconscious take over, without the conscious mind getting in the way with its doubts and fears. If the opportunity arises, take part in an art therapy class and explore your inner world in a safe, supportive environment. (See art therapy website on page 194.)

Be sure to keep a record of all achievements and accomplishments, however small, in your journal. These are ideas to get you started. If used imaginatively, journal-writing can bring a special dimension to your life and capture insights that might otherwise be overlooked or forgotten.

3. Discover Solitude

Find time regularly to be alone. You may choose to give yourself a Reiki treatment, meditate or simply be. Space such as this encourages the inner dialogue with your wiser self. Meditate by focusing on your breathing or on the flame of a candle. Alternatively, you may choose to imagine yourself being bathed in healing energy.

4. Listen to Your Dreams

Expect to receive insights in your dreams. Before drifting off to sleep, pose questions or begin to visualize the situation. Expect an answer and keep a notebook or your journal by your bed. Get into the habit of writing down your dreams as soon as you wake up, even if they seem insignificant. In time you will receive messages from your higher, wiser self and be able to recall them. Record your findings in your journal.

5. Be in the Present

Much of the day is spent living in the past or dreaming of the future. By living your life increasingly in the present, you will substantially raise your awareness. This facilitates a clearer dialogue with your inner wisdom. Spend a few moments alone, becoming more aware of all your senses. What can you hear, taste, see, feel and sense right now? Become used to tuning in to all your senses. Remember that the past has gone and the future hasn't happened. The only real time is now.

6. Make Sure You Live the Life You Want

Find out what you want to do, and then do it. Find the work you love and begin it. Visualize a positive outcome and send Reiki to energize it. Fill your life with special people and joyful experiences. As you weave magic through every part of your life, people will think you are simply lucky and have a charmed life. Little do they know that a magical life is possible for anyone who wants to make the effort. Don't wait. Your future life beckons. Go for it.

> *Go confidently in the direction of your dreams! Live the life you've imagined. As you simplify your life, the laws of the universe will be simpler.*
> HENRY DAVID THOREAU

PART FOUR

18 Your Questions Answered

In the next five chapters we focus on answering questions most often asked about Reiki training. The format is designed to provide a handy guide that can be referred to when needed.

Can Anyone Learn Reiki?

The beauty of Reiki lies in its simplicity and accessibility. Anyone who is able to attend a seminar can learn. There are no religious or cultural barriers preventing a person from being initiated. The youngest child we have taught was just 10 years old, and the most elderly person (so far) was 82. People have attended in a wheelchair. There have been participants who have been hard of hearing. A person with just one hand managed perfectly well. Our son was initiated, at his own request, at just eight years old. He did not attend a course, instead receiving attunements from us over four separate evenings.

Will Reiki Work for Me?

Yes. Everyone's ability to channel a greater amount of life-force energy is enhanced by learning Reiki. Some people have been instinctively using their own healing ability without even being aware of it, and are amazed by the increased energy flow following the attunements. Others (the majority) have never learned a healing art before, yet once their ability is awakened they discover the high frequency of life-force energy at their fingertips, and all the benefits and joy this brings.

Can You Lose the Ability to Use Reiki?

Once you are attuned, the ability to be a channel for life-force energy is available to you for the rest of your life, whether or not you choose to use it. Even after a long break you can use it without the need to attend further courses. Of course you may choose, however, to take a refresher course to refamiliarize yourself with its practice.

How Is Reiki Taught?

Reiki is taught in a group setting with others to share experiences and practise with. There are several levels, to ensure that learning is not energetically overwhelming. Courses are experiential, so there are no books to read or tests to take. It is easy to learn and classes are relaxed and enjoyable.

Could Reiki Ever Be Harmful?

No. Reiki works by dissolving barriers to harmony. It is not invasive and cannot harm. Furthermore, the energy is not given to but drawn by the recipient. It is a fine, light, high frequency that has a consciousness of its own. It is drawn to where it is needed in the quantity required. It is not possible for a person to draw 'too much'.

Do I Have to Give Up My Religious Beliefs to Learn Reiki?

No. Reiki does not interfere with any spiritual practice. It can in fact enhance it, by helping a person to become more loving and understanding, which in essence is at the heart of any spiritual tradition.

Can Reiki Be Combined with Other Healing Modalities?

While Reiki is a complete treatment, it does combine well with other complementary therapies, particularly different forms of bodywork such as reflexology, shiatsu, aromatherapy, Heller work, Rolfing and massage. Aromatherapy oils can be treated with Reiki before use. Reiki can be used for absent-healing procedures, making it a useful tool to combine with psychotherapy, hypnotherapy, counselling and coaching.

Reiki also combines well with allopathic (orthodox) medicine and medical treatments. Doctors and nurses who have taken Reiki use it to speed patients' post-operative healing. It also helps to relieve pain or anxiety in the emergency room while an uncomfortable procedure is being carried out.

We are constantly surprised by the resourcefulness of practitioners who take Reiki out to the world in their own unique way. Ben is a medical student. He is also a Second-degree Reiki practitioner. At night, like most of his peer group, he likes to socialize and frequent bars in his area. Unlike other students, Ben has come to an arrangement with the managers. They have agreed to let him offer Reiki to those who would like to try it. Together with another medical student, they have been demonstrating Reiki and offering treatments in bars and clubs on a regular basis. The noise may be loud and the atmosphere not exactly conducive, but these pioneering students have reported an enthusiastic response.

Could Reiki Improve My Sex Life?

Most definitely. Reiki opens the heart, encouraging love to flow more freely. Relationships often deepen after couples take Reiki training at the same time. Most people find that, following initiation into Reiki, they become more responsive and spontaneous. The senses become heightened. Partners with sexual issues will find it helpful to treat the genital area directly. For further information, read *Tantric Sex: How to Use Reiki to Enhance Love and Sex* by Gail Radford (Astralog).

Is It Possible to Pick Up Negative Energies from Other People?

No. Unlike some other forms of healing, you are using an external energy to give treatments, not your own. You are not affected by another person's illness or negativity, nor can they pick up yours. You are acting as a channel rather than a reservoir.

When you treat a person who is going through something you also happen to be experiencing or repressing, this could trigger off your emotions because they will have a similar frequency. For example, if you were feeling angry about something and treated someone with similar issues, you might find these feelings surfacing. This awareness may help you to deal with it and move on.

Remember, when you give a treatment you also receive one, so you might have a reaction. You may have insights into another's pain, but you won't be in a position where another's suffering becomes your own.

REIKI FIRST DEGREE

What Should Reiki First-degree Training Consist of?
Formats do vary, but most Reiki teachers familiarize students with the origins and history of Reiki. Students should receive four attunements, learning the hand positions for self-treatment and for treating others. Attunements refer to the energetic adjustment process brought about by a combination of mantras and symbols to enable a greater amount of life-force energy to flow through a person's system. The five principles are discussed, and there should be plenty of time for feedback and questions throughout the course. There should be an opportunity for each participant to give and receive a full-body treatment, as well as practising self-treatment. On the personal development side, there should be adequate support given to those with questions to ask and issues arising.

How Do I Find a Teacher Who Has Trained to a High Standard in the Usui Tradition?
This question is answered fully in Chapter 21. Briefly, it is important to determine whether a teacher has trained in the Usui system of Reiki and is someone with whom you feel you could develop a rapport. A degree of discernment may be required in order to ensure a Reiki Master is competent and able to provide you with adequate support both during and after classes.

Is There More Than One Authentic Lineage Originating from Dr Usui?
There are several authentic forms and lineages of Reiki, as Dr Usui had a number of students he worked with closely. However, not everything that calls itself Reiki actually is Reiki. Discernment is required to distinguish

the authentic forms. It may be necessary to ask searching questions to determine the origin and authenticity of a particular system.

What Kind of Support Can I Expect from a Reiki Teacher?

You should expect to be provided with a safe, supportive environment, so that you can learn and grow with joy. A supportive Reiki Master should care, listen, encourage and respect you, possibly even challenge you at times. It is important to find a teacher you feel you can trust. He or she should be able to provide adequate training without being weighed down by attachment to his or her own importance. A Master who has not dealt with the illusory nature of the ego will not be able to support others adequately.

What Can I Do If My Training Is Less than Satisfactory?

This depends on the nature of the problem. If you don't feel confident about using Reiki, you could ask your Reiki teacher if you could repeat the class. Most teachers will be happy to accommodate this request, without further charge.

If you have received the correct number of attunements, but insufficient information on the history or use of Reiki, you may be able to fill in the gaps by reading a book or doing some research on the Internet.

Students often tell us they received attunements without any other tuition. Sometimes they have not received all four of the First-degree attunements and haven't been taught to give or receive a treatment, let alone practise it. To gain the maximum benefit, you do need to know how to incorporate Reiki into your life.

If there are other reasons to believe your training was less than satisfactory, or if you feel the course itself was too superficial or energetically insubstantial, you may need to put it down to experience and retrain with an experienced Reiki Master.

After the Course, Why Do I Need to Give Myself a Treatment for 30 Days?
Initiation into Reiki raises a person's life-force energy. This can take time to assimilate. Giving yourself a treatment for a number of days following training assists this process. Physical and even emotional toxins may surface. They need releasing for healing to occur. This period of self-treatment helps a person to adjust. At the end of 30 days you will find you feel lighter, clearer and calmer.

Do I Need to Visualize or Focus on Anything to Make the Energy Flow?
No. To begin the process, place your hands on yourself or someone else, with the intent that the energy should flow. If you are treating someone else, you may wish to state that it should go to wherever it is needed, for the greatest benefit of the person concerned. During the treatment itself you will find you naturally relax into a peaceful, meditative state.

If I'm in a Hurry, Should I Just Treat the Area Most in Need?
Yes. When time is limited, place your hands directly on or over the area of discomfort. As many conditions are stress-related, treat the head positions, too. Otherwise, trust your intuitive abilities and treat areas you are drawn to.

Could Someone Feel Worse after a Reiki Treatment?
It is not usual, but it is possible. Symptoms that have been surfacing for several hours or days can materialize. When symptoms are brought to the surface like this they can be intense for a very short period, after which they usually disappear.

Sometimes, a 'healing crisis' can occur. This happens when symptoms gradually improve, only to re-occur in a sudden and dramatic way. This is usually short-lived. Very often, the condition then vanishes for ever.

19 Reiki Second Degree

How Can I Benefit from Taking a Reiki Second-degree Course?
At this level, your awareness is enhanced and you become a channel for a far greater amount of life-force energy. This enables you to give more effective treatments in a shorter space of time, and gives you the tools to direct energy to the root cause of pain and suffering – the mind.

Mental and emotional anguish often lie behind physical symptoms. By directing energy to the cause, you can become aware of limiting subconscious thought-patterns. As your awareness increases, pain diminishes.

A number of symbols are introduced at this level, which enable you to send healing energy across time and space. This may seem an extraordinary concept, but it will be explained during the course.

Symbols can be described as living energy fields. Every time they are drawn and their names pronounced, they manifest a particular frequency, each of which has a specific purpose. When used as taught, they can form an energetic pathway through which energy can be conveyed. This opens the possibility of sending energy to people and situations, as well as providing unlimited opportunities for self-healing.

One of the greatest benefits of Reiki Second Degree is the dissolving of mental and emotional blocks, allowing old thought-patterns to be completely erased. This is liberating, increasing clarity and restoring inner peace.

Once you have become accustomed to using the symbols to send energy for absent-healing, you begin to appreciate that time does not exist. You learn to send healing to difficult situations in the past and events yet to happen, in the future.

The effects of this attunement vary. Some people find their intuition is awakened or heightened after Second Degree. Others just know where to place their hands. Everyone is individual and there is no universal reaction.

To benefit fully, it is important to find a competent, experienced Usui teacher, as this level does demand a thorough explanation of the procedures, along with practical ways in which to use them. Inadequate teaching could be confusing and uninspiring, if the material is not delivered in a meaningful way. Usually, the training is lively and exciting, as the contents are both fascinating and thought-provoking.

Some Teachers Offer First- and Second-degree Courses Combined. Are These a Good Idea?

In our opinion, they are not a good idea. Each level offers a different intensity of energy and a variety of techniques. Many people have told us their combined courses were short and confusing. It takes time to assimilate each level. Furthermore, the depth of each course is sacrificed in order to cover the content. It takes time to energetically adjust, detoxify and rebalance. We suggest a minimum gap of approximately three months between study of these two different levels.

My First-degree Training Was Disappointing. How Can I Ensure that I Find the Right Teacher for Second-degree Training?

See Chapter 21 for more details of finding a teacher. Otherwise, ask for recommendations from others, go and hear a Reiki Master give a talk, or call them up. Be guided by your intuition rather than the convenience of a particular location or an inexpensive price tag. Choose the right format to gain the maximum benefit. Would a day class suit you, or would you prefer a residential course in the company of kindred spirits?

Can the Distant-healing Technique Be Used for Situations as Well as People?

Yes. It can be used to send energy not only to a number of people at the same time, but also to an unlimited number of situations. Examples are conflicts, war zones, natural disasters or wherever there is suffering or misunderstanding.

Intriguingly, it can also be used to send yourself energy. It can be sent to relationships, careers, businesses, abilities, skills and opportunities. This process of healing sent backwards and forwards in time, to past and future events, can be extraordinarily effective in bringing harmony to the present.

Energy can even be sent to objects, including cars, computers, motorcycles and electrical equipment. Of course it would be unwise to depend on repairs being carried out in this way, but it is nevertheless surprising how often it helps.

Is It OK to Send Absent Healing without Someone's Permission?

Yes. The recipient draws the energy; you cannot impose healing onto someone. With practice you can learn to sense whether a person is receiving it. If not, it won't harm them and will be available should they need it in future. The energy won't be drawn unless the person chooses to accept it. Rather like some e-mail programmes, it won't be downloaded unless the key 'open' or 'receive' is selected.

Can Reiki Be Given to Someone Who Is Terminally Ill?

Definitely. When a person's life is ending there is often the opportunity for significant healing to occur. As well as pain-relief, Reiki can bring a person closer to those around them, relieving any fear or isolation. It can help a loved one come to terms with their situation, and provide gentle and effective support. Reiki can also help replenish the energy level of the carers.

I'm Setting Up a Practice. What Should I Charge for a Reiki Treatment?

This varies depending upon where you live. As a general guide, we suggest charging about the same as a body massage in your area. Many practitioners choose to offer a discount if a series of treatments is booked. You may also wish to offer concessionary rates to students, those with disabilities and the elderly, as well as those who are financially disadvantaged.

If I Am Giving Treatments on a Regular Basis, Should I Be Insured?

While the Usui system of Reiki is not harmful in itself, we always suggest you obtain insurance if you are treating others on a professional basis. If you already practise another therapy, it is usually possible to add Reiki onto existing insurance. One way of obtaining this reasonably is by joining an organization for practitioners of complementary therapies. Most offer their members low-cost insurance. A couple are listed on page 199 of this book.

20 Master Practitioner

What Time-gap Should There Be between Second-degree and Master Practitioner Training?
The ideal gap is a minimum of three to six months. It takes time to assimilate both the energy increase and the material learned at Second Degree. Everyone is different and it's a personal decision. Some prefer to wait longer.

What Does Training at Master Practitioner Level Involve?
Training at Master Practitioner level is about mastering the self. We are often keen to help others without dealing with our own issues. This level is about finding out who you really are. It involves being able to accept and love yourself unconditionally, without being limited by the ego's illusory messages, nor deluded by attachment to your own importance.

Recognizing and integrating the different aspects of yourself liberates you from the illusion of being separated from others. Knowing we are all inter-connected, each with the capacity to be saints or sinners, can in one sense be a sobering thought. At another level, it is an exciting concept. It becomes evident that there is the seed of greatness within each of us, with the means to create our unique reality. At the very least, we can move beyond self-imposed barriers and attain freedom from limiting thought-patterns.

Master Practitioner study reflects the desire by many to train to the highest level without the responsibility of teaching. Participants learn a variety of advanced healing methods. They also receive a powerful attunement and a symbol, and ways in which to use these for healing and transformation.

Does Every Reiki Master Teach Master Practitioner?

No. It evolved out of a need by students to hold the Master energy without the responsibility of teaching. Students considering teaching Reiki often take Master Practitioner in order to integrate the energy at this level before further training. Others have no desire to teach, but wish to attain the highest practitioner level for treating others.

Will I Be Qualified to Teach Reiki after Taking Master Practitioner Training?

No. This level is not about attuning others. It is about advanced training as a practitioner and mastering the self.

How Could I Use Energy at this Level to Help Myself?

You will be able to channel a much higher frequency of energy at this level, which will release much of the denser energy in your system and raise your self-awareness. You will find yourself able to release judgement, beliefs and limitations that once held you back. The knowledge and energetic boost can help you take a more active role in creating your own experience. You will find you are able to manifest what you need to move forwards.

How Can I Use Knowledge Gained at Master Practitioner Level to Help Others?

Once you are able to move beyond limiting thought-patterns, you are also able to help others do the same. It is then possible to help them to attract positive experiences and move forward. It is beneficial to gain lots of practical experience at this stage. Offer treatments in hospices, clinics or wherever you are drawn.

21 Finding a Teacher

What Should I Look for in a Teacher or School of Reiki?
In our view it is important to find a teacher that is aligned to the Usui system. Ask if they teach Usui Reiki, or have created their own healing system. The teacher should be able to demonstrate that they offer a high standard of training. This should include personal attention during courses, plus support afterwards. It helps if you feel you have a rapport with the teacher. If possible, speak to or meet the Reiki Master before booking. At the very least, read the publicity material or find a Master who has been highly recommended by others.

What Should I Ask to Determine Whether a Reiki Master Is Right for Me?
There is some excellent tuition available, but it must be said that training as a whole is variable. It is worth investing a short amount of time and effort in assessing whether the tuition is of a high standard. We are all individual, and while there is bound to be a degree of variation in the way that Reiki is taught, it shouldn't depart too radically from the Usui system, otherwise it simply isn't Reiki.

Find out which teachers others recommend. Speak to more than one. Ask questions that determine their depth of experience. You may wish to find out what support is available after the class. Many students tell us that their Reiki Master taught a class and promptly returned to their native country. If this doesn't sound ideal for you, find a Reiki Master who is based in the country where you live. Find out what size classes are. If numbers are very large, will each participant receive enough personal attention? If you are still unsure, speak to a person or group they have taught. Ask if they are teaching purely Reiki or combining it with any other form of healing.

Ask yourself how you feel in the presence of the particular Reiki Master. Rapport is important. Do you feel this particular Reiki Master could impart information in a meaningful way? Reiki is, in essence, simplicity. Courses involve experiencing spiritual concepts and are far less concerned with intellectualizing them.

Trust your intuition. Ask questions such as 'Can you trace your lineage back to Dr Usui?' 'How long were you practising Reiki before becoming a Master?' (Hopefully, three years or longer.) 'What do you feel is your speciality as a Reiki Master?' 'How many people are there typically in your seminars?' (Classes with many more than 12 people would not allow enough time for personal attention.) Trust that the questions you need to ask will spring to mind.

What Should I Avoid?

Avoid anyone who pressures you to make a decision. Only you can decide when you would like to proceed. The Reiki Master should be a well-balanced person who is comfortable to be with. If you feel a Reiki Master tries to put you down or disrespect you in any way, look elsewhere. No matter how many degrees or qualifications a person has, you have to feel at ease in their company or it won't work. Beware of 'masters' who trained last week, having been initiated in the briefest of weekend seminars (which may have included Reiki First- and Second-degree as well!).

Avoid making decisions based on convenience. It may be worth travelling further if the Reiki Master is offering a class you are drawn to. Likewise, the cheapest option may turn out costly if, in the end, you find you have to repeat the class elsewhere.

22 Becoming a Teacher of Reiki

What Should Be My Motivation for Teaching Reiki?
Master Teacher Training is for those who wish to help others use Reiki energy for self-healing and for healing others.

The term 'Master' is used in an Eastern sense and refers to a person who has mastered the self, rather than one who has dominion over others. It is important for you to examine your reasons for wishing to train as a Reiki Master. Ensure that your motivation is not ego-based, as this can place obstacles on your own path. The objective of any spiritual practice is to gain liberation from suffering and help others to do so. Those with an inflated ego complete with grand title may not be in a position to illuminate the path for others.

How Do You Train as a Reiki Master?
Training involves becoming an understudy to an existing Reiki Master until a person is competently able to teach Reiki and assist others to benefit from its practice. Ideally, you should have been practising Reiki for a minimum of three years before considering teaching.

Unlike the other levels of Reiki, Master training is personalized on a one-to-one basis and tailored to the needs of the individual. It involves an element of co-teaching and participating in courses at all levels. Students learn how to present a workshop and understand group dynamics. Personal development skills and related spiritual disciplines unfold throughout the training. The trainee learns how to initiate others before receiving the Master's attunement.

Training involves achieving quite a number of objectives, one of which is a maturation of the personality. No one can have all the answers, but it is imperative that the trainee is equipped with the necessary tools, knowledge and spiritual understanding to guide others.

If you are considering training to be a Reiki Master, find a teacher you resonate with, as you will be spending much time with this person and need to establish a rapport, right from the start. To gain the maximum benefit, find someone you feel will take time with you and stretch you to your limit. This period should be enjoyable, challenging at times, and ultimately rewarding.

Should Reiki Master Training Be Taught as a Seminar?

Opinions vary. It is possible to learn how to attune people in a single weekend. but not possible to learn how to guide them. The best way to learn is on a one-to-one basis. In this way, the training can be personalized to the needs of the student. At this level it is important that the student receives all the necessary attention in order to learn, grow and assimilate the appropriate information. A seminar alone cannot provide this.

I'm a Reiki Master, Yet My Training Only Lasted for a Weekend and I Don't Feel I Have Enough Knowledge to Teach Others – What Can I Do?

We are often asked this question. There are a number of choices. Contact the Reiki Master who initiated you and discuss your uncertainties. They may be able to help. Find out if you can take part in extra seminars, both as a student and as a trainee teacher. This will give you the opportunity to ask additional questions and gain further experience.

If your initiating Master is not available or has left the country, you may find the information you seek in books or on the Internet. If this does not solve the problem, you may need to consider retraining elsewhere.

Master Teacher Training – Is It for Me?

Only you can decide. If you strongly aspire to teach others, you will find this is an extraordinary path for healing and awakening. The effects of spending so much time in the energy, with the responsibility of teaching and attuning, bring many gifts. You find yourself becoming closer to the source of your own being.

One day when you are teaching, you may look around and suddenly notice that every person in the room is a different part of you. Suddenly you will know that there aren't any Masters or students. Just a group of people who have come together to remember who they truly are. When this happens, you will experience the oneness of all. From this place of knowing the view is spectacular and you will truly be a great teacher.

> *You cannot teach a man anything*
> *You can only help him to find it within himself.*
> GALILEO

PART FIVE

Going Further with Reiki

When I was young and free and my imagination had no limits
I dreamed of changing the world.
As I grew older and wiser, I discovered the world would not
  change
So I shortened my sights somewhat and decided to change only
  my country.
But it too seemed immovable.
As I grew into my twilight years, in one last desperate attempt
I settled for changing only family, those closest to me
But alas, they would have none of it.
And now as I lay on my deathbed, I suddenly realise:
If I had only changed myself first
Then, by example I would have changed my family.
From their inspiration and encouragement,
I would then have been able to better my country
And who knows, I may even have changed the world

ANONYMOUS (TAKEN FROM A TOMBSTONE AT WESTMINSTER
ABBEY)

Reiki can open hearts and minds to infinite possibilities. This healing energy can be said to equate to unconditional love, which transcends all barriers to transform even the most difficult situation. Jimi Hendrix was once quoted as saying, 'When the power of love overcomes the love of power, the world will know peace.'

In this book we have provided some tools and strategies that you can use for healing and transformation. Once you get to grips with the concept that thought is creative, you can have great fun attracting or manifesting whatever you need in your life, from parking spaces to more clients, from friendships to love, from the perfect job to the perfect home. Through the power of love and the power of thought, who knows what we might be capable of?

Reiki is an incredibly versatile, though simple, spiritual practice. It aligns you to your highest energetic frequency so that you can receive the greatest guidance of all: your own inner wisdom.

It is our wish that you will find creative ways of using Reiki to transform your life, so that you can enjoy every moment to the fullest. And when you start to experience this healing in your life, let us know by letter or e-mail, so that we can share your joy (our address is on page 189).

Your thoughts, your words, your actions are the tools with which you can manifest your reality. So, bring a little magic into your life and make your life extraordinary.

Wishing you joy, success and many incredible experiences.

In love, light and peace,

Chris and Penny Parkes

Chris and Penny's Reiki Lineage

Dr Mikao Usui
Dr Chujiro Hayashi
Hawayo Takata
Barbara Weber Ray
John Latz
Clarity Ann Martin
Carrlyn Clay

Chris and Penny welcome questions and feedback from readers. All letters and e-mails will be replied to, although sometimes this may take time due to their travel commitments. They can be contacted at:

The Reiki School
Budworth
Shay Lane
Hale
Altrincham
WA15 8UE

0161 980 6453
Fax: 0161 980 6972
e-mail: info@thereikischool.co.uk
website: www.thereikischool.co.uk

The Reiki School can also supply treatment tables and CDs adapted for Reiki treatments and relaxation.

Using Hypnotherapy with Reiki

Here is an example of a hypnotherapy script which could be used for IBS. It is ideal to listen to while giving yourself a Reiki treatment. You can change, personalize and adapt it in any way you choose.

Allow yourself to relax and become comfortable ... In a moment I am going to count down from three to one ... and ask that you place your hands on your stomach ... OK ... three ... two ... one ... and now place your hands on your stomach ... as your hands rest on your stomach ... you'll begin to feel a warmth spreading out around the muscles in this area ... feel the warmth as it spreads out releasing any tension ... relaxing you more and more ...

As your hands remain in this position, they will become warmer and warmer ... feel the warmth as the energy flows ... healing and nurturing ... warming and soothing ... calming and relaxing your stomach ...

As you feel this healing glow ... you know that your unconscious mind is directing all your inner resources to the areas you need it most ... know too, that Reiki energy will be flowing through to where it is needed ... calming ... healing ... and soothing ... as you relax more and more ...

Your thoughts and feelings affect the muscles of the gut ... and it follows that you are able to control the gut muscles ... easily

... whenever you like ... you can remove pain ... remove bloating ... remove discomfort ... and normalize your bowel movements ... to your own satisfaction.

Whenever you place your hands on your stomach ... you will be able to control the muscles ... you will feel the same sense of warmth and comfort that you feel now ... and by placing your hands in this same position ... it will act as a signal for your subsconscious mind ... for you ... to take control of the muscles in your gut ... to remove bloating ... remove discomfort and normalize your bowel movement to your own satisfaction.

Imagine you are lying beside a beautiful river in the heart of the countryside ... hear the sounds of the flowing water ... picture the calm, clear water ... tranquil, rhythmic ... and orderly ... no rushing ... no delays ... no hurry ... just a steady ... peaceful rhythmic flow ... just a calm, steady flow ... normal movement ... through your gut ... as you relax more and more.

Visualize the energy as it flows from your hands ... feel the strength of your mind, because the stronger your mind ... the more and more control you will acquire ... no pain ... no bloating ... no discomfort ... you can achieve this ... you can ... and you will ... soon you will hardly be aware that you have a stomach ... it's working so well ... so normally ... so steadily.

Feel another surge of energy ... as the warmth spreads ... indicating that you are in control of your gut ... healing ... soothing ... wherever you are ... at any time ... in any place.

Bibliography and Further Reading

M Ali, *Integrated Health Bible* (Vermilion, 2001)

BMA *Complete Family Health Guide* (Dorling Kindersley, 2000)

Deepak Chopra, *Quantum Healing: Exploring the Frontiers of Mind–Body Healing* (Bantam, 1989)

T Dethlefsen and R Dahlke, *The Healing Power of Illness* (Vega Books, 2002)

M Fennell, *Overcoming Low Self-esteem* (Constable & Robinson, 1999)

B Flaws, *Hay Fever* (Foulsham, 2000)

Louise Hay, *Heal Your Body* (Hay House, 1999)

J Hillman, *The Soul's Code* (Transworld Publishers, 1997)

P Holford, *The Optimum Nutrition Bible* (Piatkus Books, 1998)

Dr J Oschman, *Energy Medicine: The Scientific Basis* (Churchill Livingstone, 2000)

C and P Parkes, *Reiki: The Essential Guide to the Ancient Healing Art* (Vermilion, 1998)

Dr R Sharma, *The Family Encyclopaedia of Health: A Guide to Integrated Medicine* (HarperCollins, 2002)

B and F Stiene, *The Reiki Sourcebook* (O Books, 2003)

A Weil, *Spontaneous Healing* (Time-Warner Paperbacks, 1995)

------, Ask Dr Weil: *Common Illnesses* (Time-Warner Paperbacks, 1999)

L Whitworth, *Co-Active Coaching* (Davies-Black Publishing, 1999)

Reading for Inspiration

W Dyer, *There is a Spiritual Solution to Every Problem* (HarperCollins, 2002)

G Edwards, *Living Magically* (Piatkus, 1999)

------, *Pure Bliss* (Piatkus, 2000)

F Harrold, *Be Your Own Life Coach* (Hodder Mobius, 2001)

------, *The Ten Minute Life Coach* (Hodder Mobius, 2002)

L Hay, *You Can Heal Your Life* (Hay House, 2002)

R Holden, *Happiness Now!* (Hodder Mobius, 1999)

P Horan, *Empowerment Through Reiki* (Lotus Press, 1992)

------, *Reiki: 108 Questions & Answers* (Full Circle Publishing, 1998)

M Lambert, *An Introduction to Reiki: Healing Energy for Mind, Body & Spirit* (Collins & Brown, 2000)

------, *Clearing the Clutter: 100 Ways to Energise Your Life* (Cico Books, 2001)

J Redfield, *The Celestine Prophecy* (Bantam, 1994)

C Richardson, *Take Time for Your Life* (Bantam, 2000)

A Robbins, *Unlimited Power* (Pocket Books, 2001)

-------, *Awaken the Giant Within* (Pocket Books, 2001)

N D Walsch, *Conversations with God: An Uncommon Dialogue* (Hodder Mobius, 1997)

D Walter, *Go for It!* (Quadrille Publishing, 2003)

S Wilde, *Infinite Self* (Hay House, 1996)

Books for Superhealth

S Clark, *What Really Works: The Insider's Guide to Natural Health* (HarperCollins, 2003)

Dr P D'Adamo, *Eat Right for Your Type* (Century, 2001)

------, *Live Right for Your Type* (Penguin, 2002)

M Hall, *Reiki for Common Ailments* (Piatkus, 1999)

P Holford, *Supplements for Super Health* (Piatkus, 2000)

L Kenton, *The X-Factor Diet* (Vermilion, 2002)

E Mindell, *The Vitamin Bible* (Arlington Books, 1985)

------, *Earl Mindell's Diet Bible* (Fair Winds Press, 2003)

J Sarno, *Healing Back Pain* (Little, Brown & Company, 1997)

A Weil, *Eight Weeks to Optimum Health* (Time-Warner Paperbacks, 1997)

Useful Websites and Addresses

Coaching, Counselling and Psychological Therapies

American Art Therapy Association
www.arttherapy.org

British Association for Counselling and Psychotherapy
www.bacp.co.uk

British Association of Art Therapists
www.baat.org

British Psychological Society
www.bps.org.uk

National College of Hypnosis and Psychotherapy
www.hypnotherapyuk.net

Relate
www.relate.org.uk

Stephen Haynes, Clairvoyant Life Guide
www.selfpower.com
01263 722 257

The Business Coaching Company
www.thebusinesscoachingco.com

The Coaching Academy
www.lifecoachingacademy.com

Health and Nutrition

ABC Homeopathy
www.abchomeopathy.com

American Association of Oriental Medicine
www.aaom.org

BBC Online Health and Fitness
www.bbc.co.uk/health

Bernie Siegel The Mind–Body Wellness Centre
www.mind-body.org

Bristol Cancer Care Clinic
www.bristolcancerhelp.org

British Acupuncture Council
www.acupuncture.org.uk

Dr Andrew Weil
www.drweilselfhealing.com

Dr Mosaraf Ali
www.dr-ali.co.uk

Dr Peter D'Adamo
www.dadamo.com

Feldenkrais Guild UK
www.feldenkrais.co.uk

Health Supplement Information Service
www.hsis.org

Hypnotherapy Home Audio Courses
www.ibsaudioprogram.com

Kailash Centre of Oriental Medicine
www.orientalhealing.co.uk

Kombucha Tea
www.sulis-health.co.uk/kombucha/network.shtml

Leslie Kenton
www.lesliekenton.com

Patrick Holford
www.patrickholford.com

Psychocalisthenics
www.pcals.com

Register of Chinese Herbal Medicine
www.rchm.co.uk

Self Help UK
www.self-help.org.uk

Trager UK
www.trager.co.uk or www.trager.com

Viniyoga
www.viniyoga.co.uk

World Health Organization
www.who.int

Reiki

Australian Reiki Connection Inc.
www.australianreikiconnection.com.au

International Association of Reiki Professionals (USA)
www.iarp.org

International House of Reiki
www.reiki.net.au

The International Institute of Reiki Training (Australia)
www.taoofreiki.com

The Reiki Alliance (Worldwide)
www.reikialliance.com

The Reiki Association (UK)
www.reikiassociation.org.uk

The Reiki Federation (UK)
www.reikifed.co.uk

The Reiki School (UK)
www.thereikischool.co.uk

Centres for Holistic Treatments

The Hale Clinic (London)
www.haleclinic.com

Violet Hill Studios (Centre for Healing Arts) (London)
www.violethillstudios.com

Vitamin and Mineral Supplements

Nature's Best
www.naturesbest.com

The Nutri Centre
www.nutricentre.com

Revital
www.revital.com

Eco-friendly Painting and Decorating

Bioshield (US)
www.bioshieldpaint.com

Ecos Organic Paints (UK)
www.ecospaints.com

Insurance for Practitioners of Complementary Therapies

H & L Balen & Co
33 Graham Road
Great Malvern
Worcestershire WR14 2HU
01684 893006
website: www.balen.co.uk

Independent Professional Therapists International
8 Ordsall Road
Retford
Nottinghamshire DN22 7PL
01777 700383
e-mail: enquiries@iptuk.com
website: www.iptiuk.com

Complementary Therapy Organizations

UK

British Complementary Medical Association
PO Box 5122
Bournemouth BH8 0WG
0845 345 5977
e-mail: membership@bcma.co.uk
website: www.bcma.co.uk

Complementary Medical Association
67 Eagle Heights
The Falcons
Bramlands Close
London SW11 2IJ
Tel/Fax: 0845 129 8434
e-mail: info@the-cma.org.uk
website: www.the-cma.org.uk

International Guild of Professional Practitioners
4 Heathfield Terrace
Chiswick
London W4 4JE
020 8994 7856
Fax: 020 8994 7880
e-mail: professionals@itecworld.co.uk
website: www.igpp.co.uk

US

American Holistic Health Association
PO Box 17400
Anaheim, CA 92817-7400
(714) 779-6152
e-mail: mail@ahha.org
website: www.ahha.org

Index

15-Minute Tai Chi

STRONG BODY, STILL MIND

Master John Ding
with Dr Alan Ding

Whatever your age or level of fitness, Tai Chi is the ultimate form of exercise to keep you strong and healthy in body and mind. Master John Ding has specially developed a shortened form of Tai Chi, so that even the busiest person can fully benefit from all that Tai Chi has to offer. With just 15 minutes' practice a day you can:

- Improve flexibility, posture and balance
- Speed up recovery from illness, injury and surgery
- Sleep more soundly and enjoy new levels of energy
- Manage stress and prevent and resolve conflict
- Boost immunity and counteract the effects of ageing
- Lower blood pressure and prevent heart disease.

Suitable even for the complete novice, this clear and practical book makes Tai Chi fully compatible with contemporary busy lifestyles.

Master John Ding is the 6th Generation Yang Style Tai Chi Chuan. He is the founder of the John Ding International Academy of Tai Chi Chuan, and gives regular Tai Chi courses and seminars. **Dr Alan Ding**, 7th Generation, Yang Style Tai Chi Chuan, is a qualified physician and chief instructor of the academy.

15-Minute Yoga

YOGA FOR A BUSY WORLD

Godfrey Devereux

Yoga is the perfect form of exercise, bringing mind and body together to benefit every aspect of your life and health. Practising for just 15 minutes a day will:

- Work every muscle in the body
- Flush and cleanse every blood vessel
- Calm the nerves and relax the mind
- Massage the brain
- Realign bones and improve posture
- Enhance skin quality
- Focus attention and improve concentration
- Generate energy and create vitality

Now there is no need to compromise your schedule to practise yoga. This book contains six different 15-minute yoga routines that are simple, easy to learn, effective and safe. Detailed instruction in the form, movement, breathing and concentration methods are given for each posture, and the six sequences offer a balanced range of effects which will satisfy the changing demands of even the busiest lifestyle.

These routines have been developed by **Godfrey Devereux**, the creator of the Dynamic Yoga Method. Formerly Director of Yoga at The Life Centre in London, he now runs a Yoga Training Centre in Ibiza, Spain.

Practical Reiki

A STEP-BY-STEP GUIDE

Mari Hall

Practical Reiki is a fully illustrated, complete guide to Reiki, the universal, life-giving energy system. Reiki is a way of transferring energy by laying on hands, and can bring great relief, not just to the physical body, but also on an emotional, mental and spiritual level. Comprehensive and straightforward, *Practical Reiki* shows how you can benefit from this ancient art and learn to use Reiki on yourself, on others and even on your animals. Discover:

- The spiritual principles of Reiki
- Self-treatment
- Treating others
- Reiki and the emotions
- Using Reiki in conjunction with other healing methods
- The endocrine system and the chakras

'Mari Hall once again shows her skill and compassion in this precise and down-to-earth book.' *Janeanne Narrin*

Mari Hall founded and directs the International Association of Reiki and is a dedicated Reiki Master Teacher. She is also the author of *Reiki for the Soul*.

Make
www.thorsonselement.com
your online sanctuary

Get online information, inspiration and
guidance to help you on the path to physical
and spiritual well-being. Drawing on the integrity
and vision of our authors and titles, and with
health advice, articles, astrology, tarot, a
meditation zone, author interviews and events
listings, www.thorsonselement.com is a great
alternative to help create space and peace
in our lives.

So if you've always wondered about practising
yoga, following an allergy-free diet, using the
tarot or getting a life coach, we can point you
in the right direction.

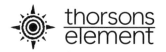

thorsons
element